The Mind Diet Cookbook

The Best Recipes to Keep Your Brain Healthy

BY: Ivy Hope

Copyright © 2020 by Ivy Hope

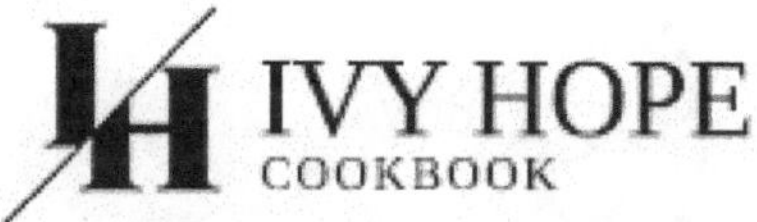

Copyright/License Page

Table of Contents

Introduction

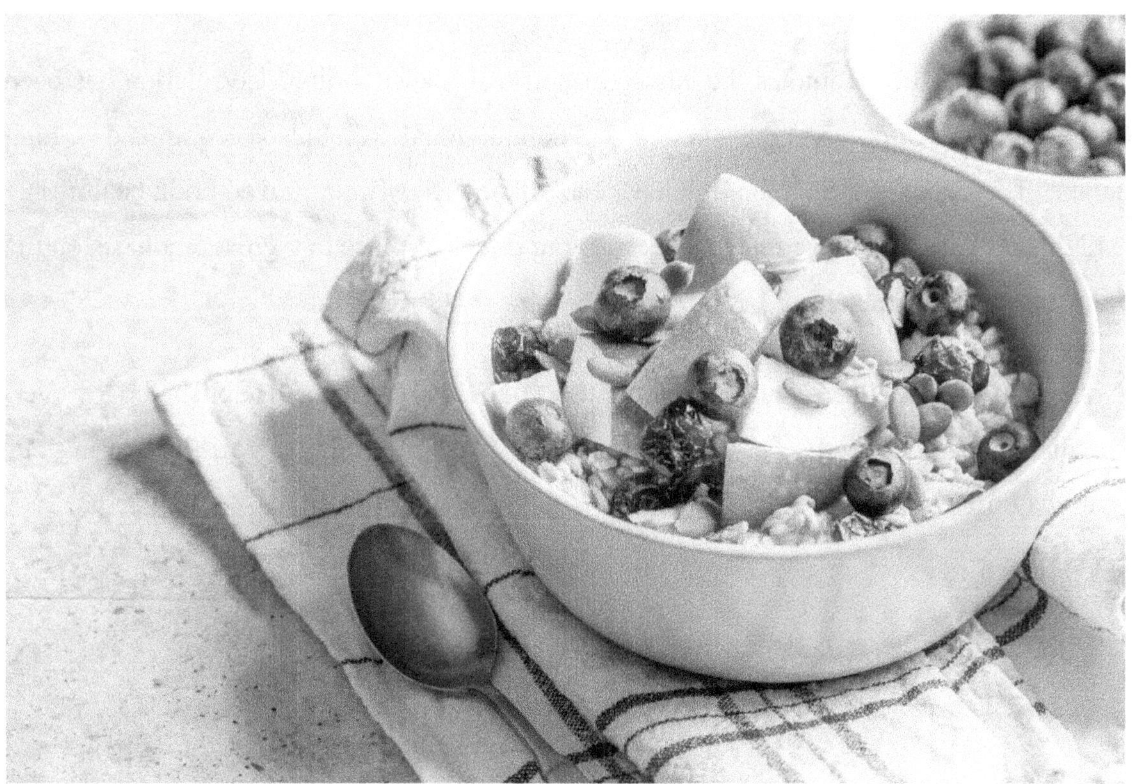

What Is the MIND Diet?

Experts have reviewed the combination of the DASH and Mediterranean diets as a powerful and potent regime. Studies have revealed that these diets have positively impacted several chronic diseases including but not limited to lowered blood pressure, reduced risk of heart disease and diabetes.

To specifically target improved brain function and prevent dementia, researchers created a diet for this purpose. To make this possible, they combined concepts from the Mediterranean and DASH diets that were proven to increase the brain's function.

This combined diet promotes the eating of berries because a direct correlation has been associated with improved brain functions. The individuals' diet also recommends a high intake of fruits, even though no link has been established with improved brain health. The MIND diet encourages the intake of berries but does not place any great emphasis on the intake of fruit in general.

No structured guideline on how to follow the MIND diet has been established. However, the diet encourages the use of certain foods and discourages the use of Five (5) in your everyday life.

Top 10 foods for improving cognitive performance

The MIND diet encourages intake 10 following foods:

Beans:

This food should be included in at least four meals per week. This diet recommends all beans, peas, lentils and soybeans.

Berries:

This food should be included in at least two meals per week. Even though published research only refers to strawberries, but other berries such as blueberries, raspberries, and blackberries, should be incorporated into their antioxidant benefits.

Fish:

This food should be included at least once per week. Try using fish that contains high amounts of omega-3 fatty acids like sardines, salmon, mackerel, trout, or tuna.

Green leafy vegetables:

Try to consume at least 6 servings of green leafy vegetables weekly. This includes salads kale, spinach, and cooked greens. Other vegetable types should be used daily in addition to these vegetables. Non-starchy vegetables are more suitable because they contain a lot of nutrients and are low in calories.

Nuts:

Try to consume a minimum of 5 servings of nuts per week. A variety of nuts should be included.

Olive oil:

This food should be used as your main cooking oil.

Poultry:

This food should be included in at least twice per week. Fried chicken is not encouraged with this diet.

Whole grains:

This food should be included in at least three servings per day. Include whole grains like quinoa, oatmeal, brown rice, 100% whole-wheat bread and whole-wheat pasta.

Wine:

Both red and white wine can benefit the brain's health. However, most researchers focus on the resveratrol compound found in red wine, which can fight against Alzheimer's disease. Aim for no more than one glass day.

Other Veggies

Around one serving per day, including leafy greens, the MIND diet (along with every balanced diet) emphasizes vegetables and seeks a different veggie form every day. It doesn't have to be difficult. Place tomatoes and red pepper strips in sandwiches and fry them with broccoli, cauliflower, bring nice veggie noodles into pasta dinners (such as zucchini or carrot noodles) or just snack them with cherry tomatoes and hummus.

Here's what the MIND diet will limit:

1. Red Meat

Red meat has more fat than other sources of protein, such as poultry or tofu. One study also combined an increase in brain iron with an increased risk of Alzheimer's and suggested that high red meat intake could be a factor.

2. Fried and Fast Food

Many fried foods have unhealthy saturated fat levels, as do other fast foods.

3. Whole-Fat Cheese

Take not more than a single serving/week. Cheese saturated fat is high. While you might have learned that processed cheese containing the metal aluminum may increase the risk of dementia, in recent years, it has been refuted that trace quantity of aluminum from food increases the risk of Alzheimer's.

4. Butter /Margarine

Not more than one tablespoon/day. Butter is high in saturated fat, while vegetable oil, such as soybean oil for omega-6 fats, contains margarine. Too many omega-6s fats can cause inflammation to increase.

5. Pastries and Sweets

A maximum of five servings/week. These treats are also high in saturated fat and sugar. Sugar can also activate the recompense mechanism of your body, which makes you crave for more.

Breakfast Recipes

If you have to stick to a healthy feeding program, then you should have a proper choice of foods to take. The meals here are special to suit all your breakfast needs. Each recipe has its own unique ingredients that carry nutritional benefits. Therefore, the meals are energizing and healthy when you start with them in the morning. Check them out and enjoy

Peanut Butter and Chocolate Smoothie

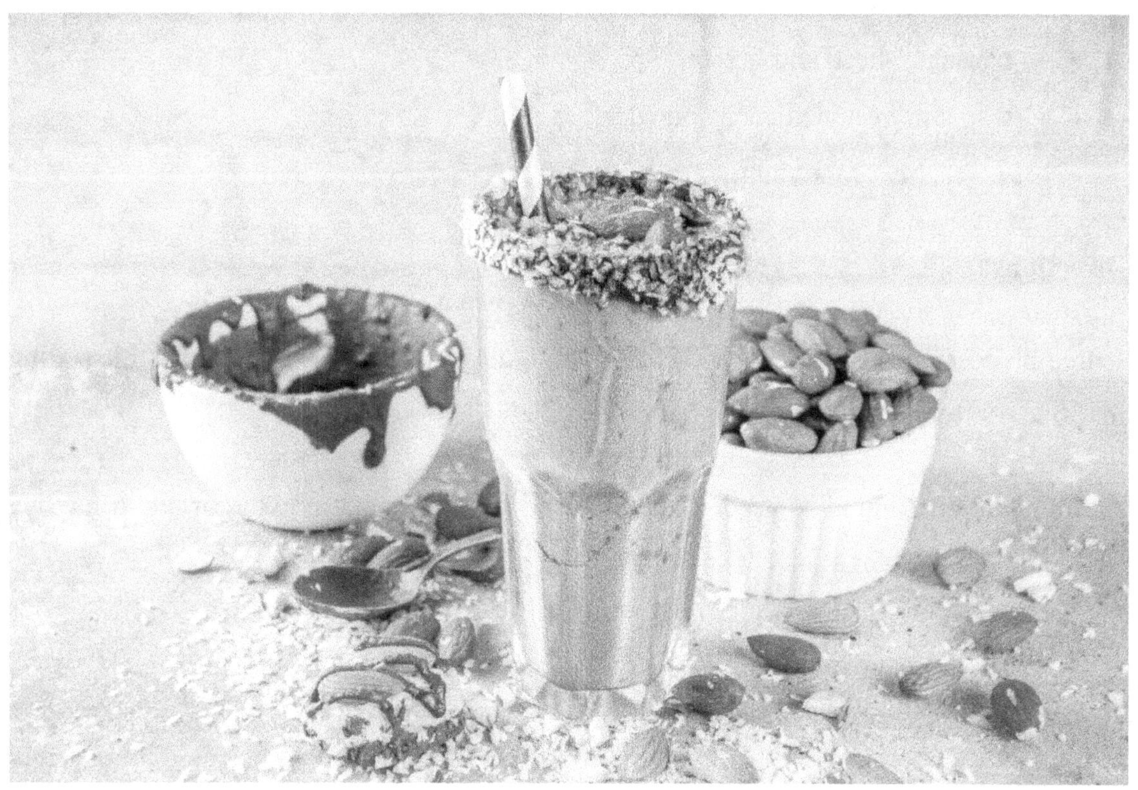

The smoothie is loaded with all the nutrients that will serve well all the health needs of your body and packed with many benefits and it is an essential way to start your morning.

Servings: 4

Cook time: 25 minutes

Ingredients:

- 2 c. vanilla nondairy milk
- 4 bananas, sliced and frozen
- 1 tbsp. unsweetened cocoa powder
- ½ c. creamy peanut butter

Directions:

1. In a blender, blend all the ingredients on high until smooth, or on the smoothie setting for 30 to 60 seconds.

2. Add additional liquid as needed and re-blend for a thinner smoothie or add a few ice cubes and re-blend for a thicker smoothie.

3. Serve chilled.

Mozzarella and Zucchini Frittata

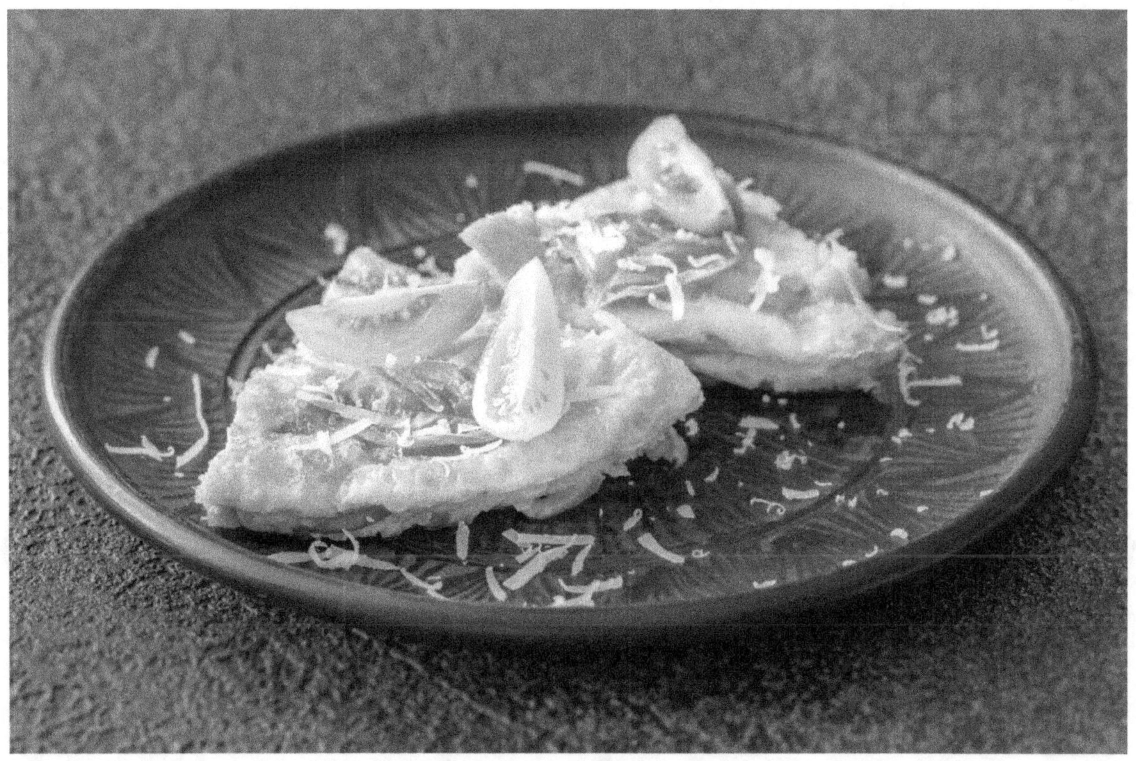

Versatility is part of what you will gain from a frittata. With a combination of mozzarella and other essential ingredients, you will enjoy your morning especially when you have a busy day ahead.

Servings: 4

Cook time: 3 minutes

Ingredients

- 2 tbsp. extra virgin olive oil
- ½ c. fresh basil
- ¼ tsp. pepper
- 1 zucchini
- 7 large eggs, beaten
- 2/3 c. fresh mozzarella
- ½ tsp. salt
- ½ red onion
- ¼ lb. cremini mushrooms
- 1 tsp. turmeric

Directions

1. Slice the red onion thinly. Slice the mushroom and zucchini. Dice the mozzarella.

2. Preheat oven to 350 degrees F. Sauté mushrooms, zucchini and onion in oil until soft; transfer to shallow baking dish.

3. Whisk turmeric, salt, pepper, and eggs; pour over zucchini mixture.

4. Bake for about 3 minutes or until eggs are set.

5. Sprinkle basil and mozzarella on top; return to oven.

6. When eggs are done, remove from oven. Slice and enjoy!

Spinach and Egg Bites

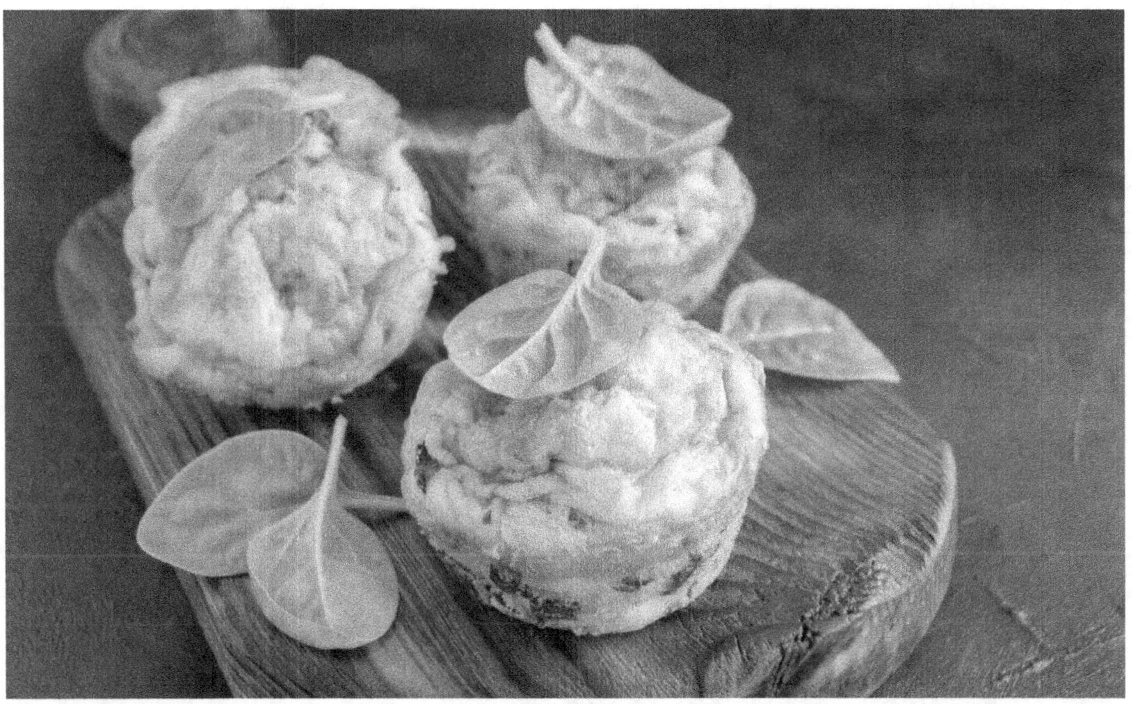

It is sometimes difficult to establish the perfect, quick and easy meal that can prepare you for the day. But a customizable meal like Spinach and Egg Bites should serve you well before doing any other thing. The meal is packed with a range of nutritious ingredients that will cater to your health needs.

Servings: 4

Cook time: 12 minutes

Ingredients

- 1 tsp. turmeric
- ½ tsp. salt
- 1 c. spinach, roughly chopped
- 2 c. shitake mushrooms, chopped
- 1/3 c. green onions, chopped
- ½ c. nutritional yeast
- 6 eggs
- ½ c. uncooked millet
- 2 c. water
- 1 large clove garlic, peeled and pressed
- 1 c. coconut milk
- ½ tsp. pepper

Directions

1. Preheat the oven to 350 degrees F. Oil muffin tins.

2. Using a medium pot, set over medium high heat, toast in the millet as you stir occasionally.

3. Add salt and water. Increase the heat and allow to boil while covered. Slightly lower the intensity of the heat to continue cooking until the water is completely absorbed.

4. In a bowl, whisk pepper, eggs, salt, turmeric, coconut milk, and garlic. Toss in mushrooms, green onions, spinach, and millet.

5. Spoon the mixture into muffin cups; bake for 12 minutes.

6. Once the egg bites are removed from oven, sprinkle with nutritional yeast. Let cool slightly

7. before you serve.

Breakfast Burrito

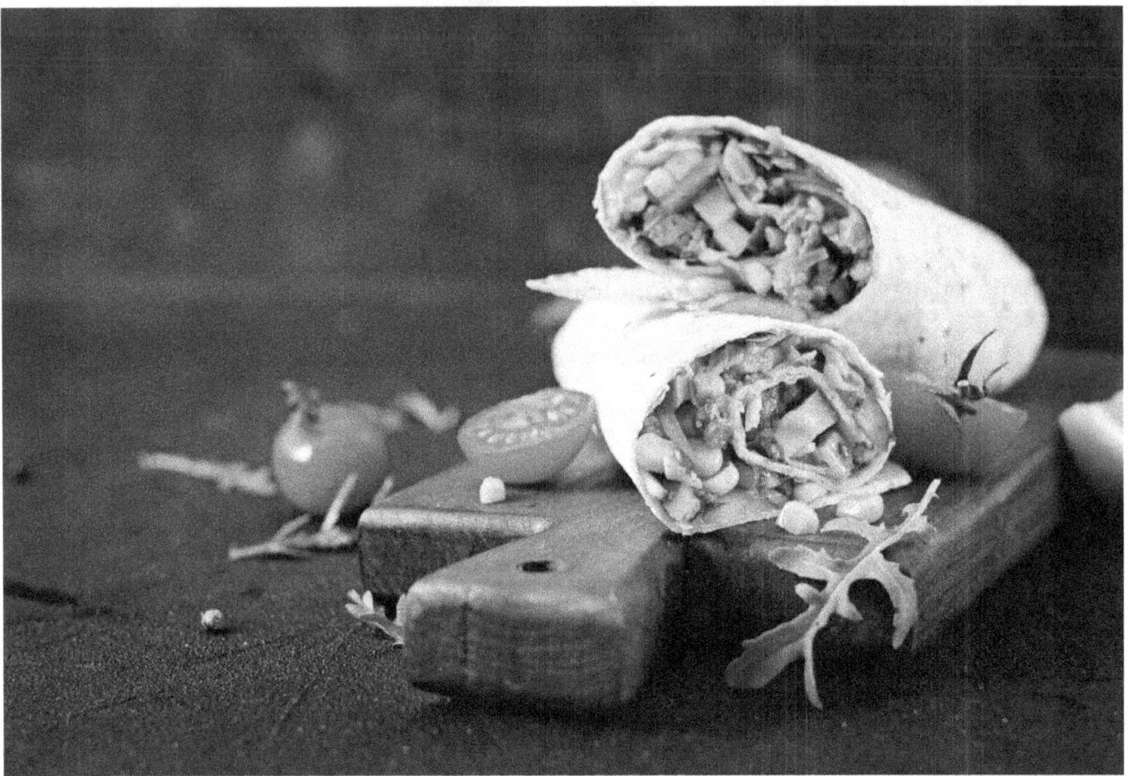

A busy day ahead needs the best starter. Breakfast Burrito is the exact option for starting your morning in a cheerful way. With a range of perfectly chosen and healthy ingredients, you can be sure of being strong all through the day.

Servings: 4

Cooking time: 6 minutes

Ingredients

- ½ lb. ground bison
- ½ c. sour cream (optional)
- 10 eggs
- 1 c. mushrooms
- ½ tsp. Himalayan salt
- 1 tsp. pepper
- 2 cloves garlic
- 1 avocado
- 1 lime
- 2 tbsp. olive oil
- ¼ c. cilantro
- 1 bunch green onions
- 1 tsp. turmeric
- ½ tsp. cumin

Directions

1. Separate eggs and put whites in one bowl and yolks in another.

2. Chop green onions, mushrooms, and cilantro.

3. Peel and press or finely mince garlic. Peel and dice avocado. Slice lime into wedges. Stirring frequently, brown buffalo in oil over medium heat, crumbling meat as it cooks.

4. Add in green onions, garlic, turmeric, and cumin. When the meat is mostly cooked, add mushrooms and continue to cook, stirring frequently, until they are soft.

5. Stir in egg yolks and cook until set. Meanwhile, whisk egg whites, season with salt and pepper. Pour a quarter of the mixture into a lightly oiled skillet or omelet pan.

6. Cook very gently over low heat for about thirty seconds, then cover and cook for a minute more. Slide the egg white "tortillas" onto a plate.

7. Roll egg mixture into the tortillas, garnish with avocado, parsley, and a squeeze of lime.

8. Serve with a dollop of sour cream, if desired

Mocha-Banana Smoothie

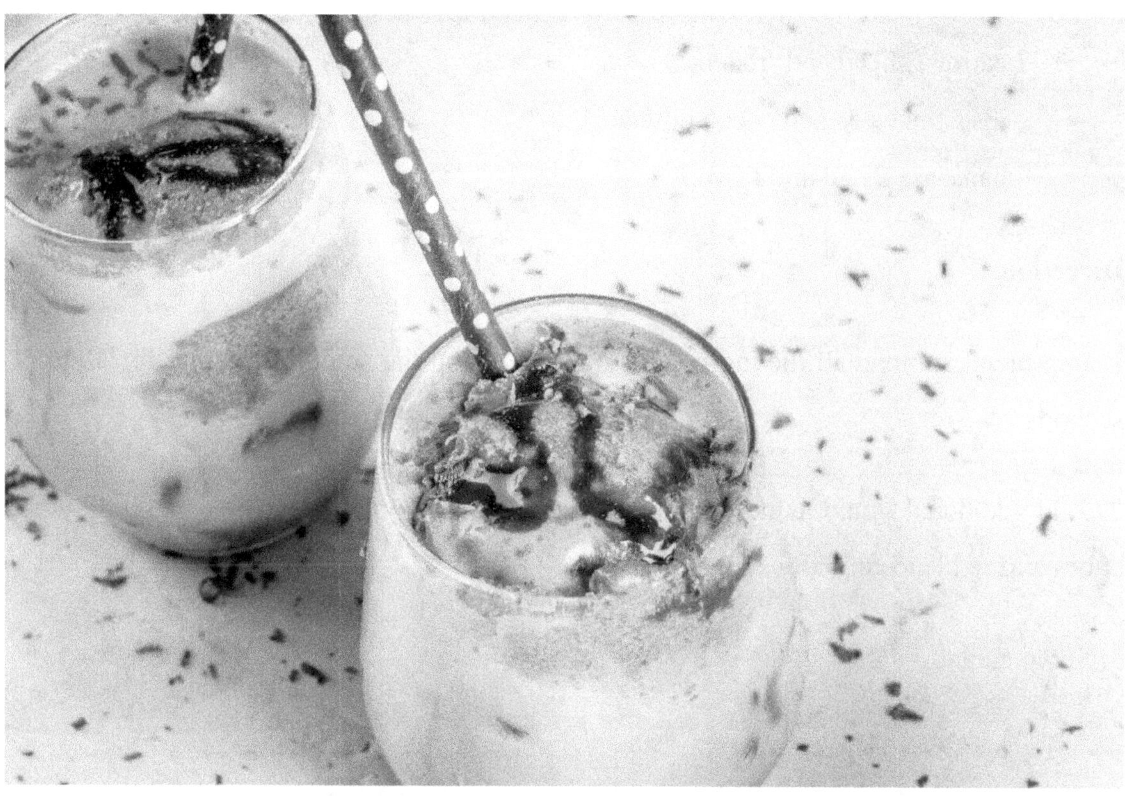

Just a simple addition of measured amount of carrots adds substance to the smoothie. It takes a shorter time to prepare. All is done just with a few ingredients. Enjoy the smoothie!

Servings: 4

Cook time: 5 minutes

Ingredients:

- 2 c. brewed coffee, chilled
- 2 carrots, sliced and frozen
- 2 tbsp. unsweetened cocoa powder
- 4 bananas, sliced and frozen

Directions:

1. In a blender, blend all the ingredients on high, or on the smoothie setting for 30 to 60 seconds.

2. Add additional liquid as needed and re-blend for a thinner smoothie or add a few ice cubes and re-blend for a thicker smoothie.

3. Serve chilled.

Overnight oats

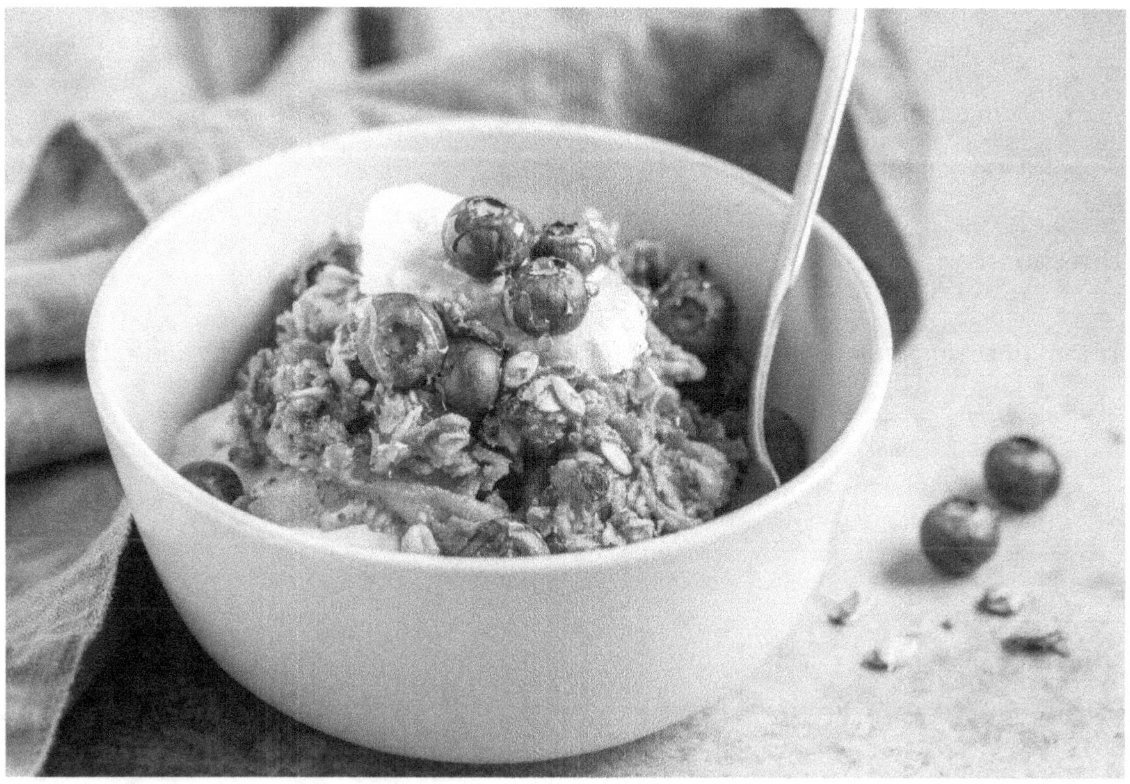

With a simple way of preparation, all you need is to pack a few essential ingredients in a sizeable jar, cover it and refrigerate overnight. It is a wonderful meal to prepare ahead for busy mornings.

Servings: 3

Cook time: 3 minutes

Ingredients:

- 1 c. almond milk.
- ½ c. blueberries berries
- ½ c. rolled oats.
- 1 tsp. vanilla.

Directions:

1. Put all the ingredients in an 8-ounce jar and Stir. Place lid on the jar and refrigerate overnight.

Quiche

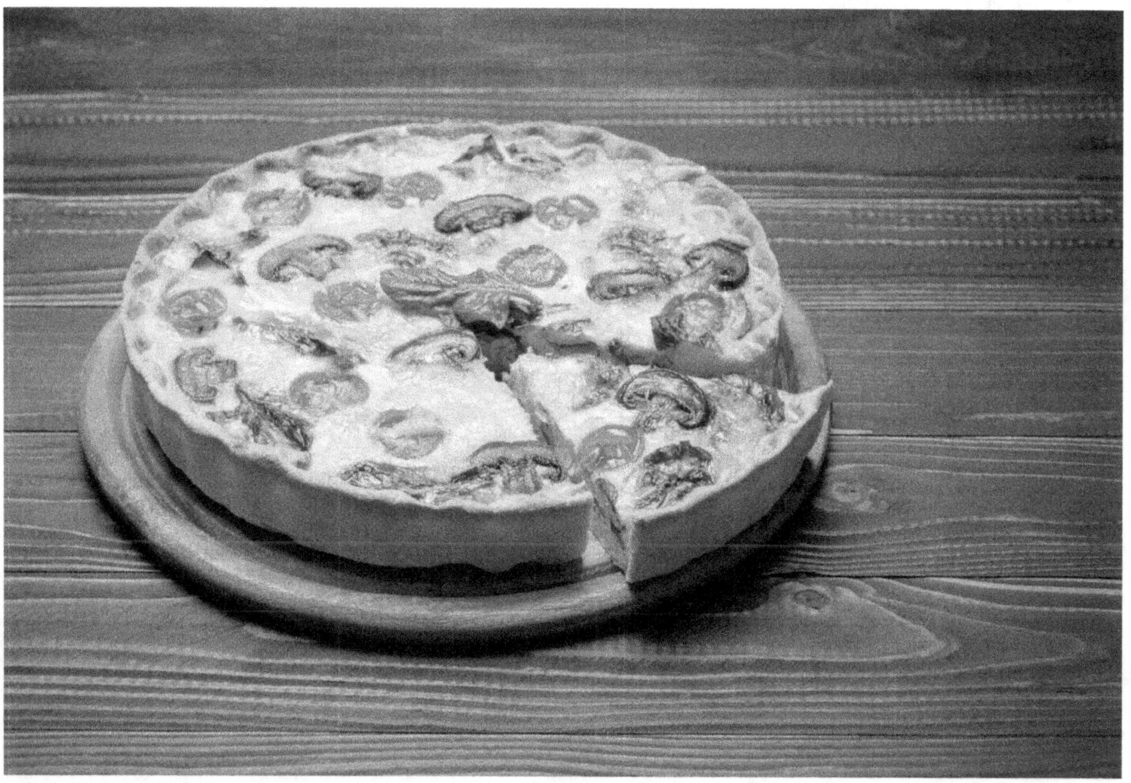

All you will need to use is a combination of mushrooms, onion, cheese, fresh spinach and scrambled eggs. In about half an hour, you will be ready to start your day in a perfect way.

Servings: 4

Cook time: 30 minutes

Ingredients:

- 4 eggs, scrambled.
- Olive oil
- 1 c. fresh spinach.
- ¼ c. grated cheese.
- ½ c. chopped onions.
- ½ c. sliced mushrooms.

Directions:

1. Preheat the oven to 350 ° F. Set a 9-inch pie pot in place.

2. Pour ample olive oil into the pot to avoid sticking vegetables. Add onions and mushrooms, fry over low heat, and stir until the onions are slightly translucent and mushrooms begin to change color. Add in spinach and stir. Add in the eggs and cheese and blend well.

3. Place in the saucepan.

4. Bake for ½ hour at 350 degrees F or until the toothpick inserted comes out dry.

Scrambled Tofu

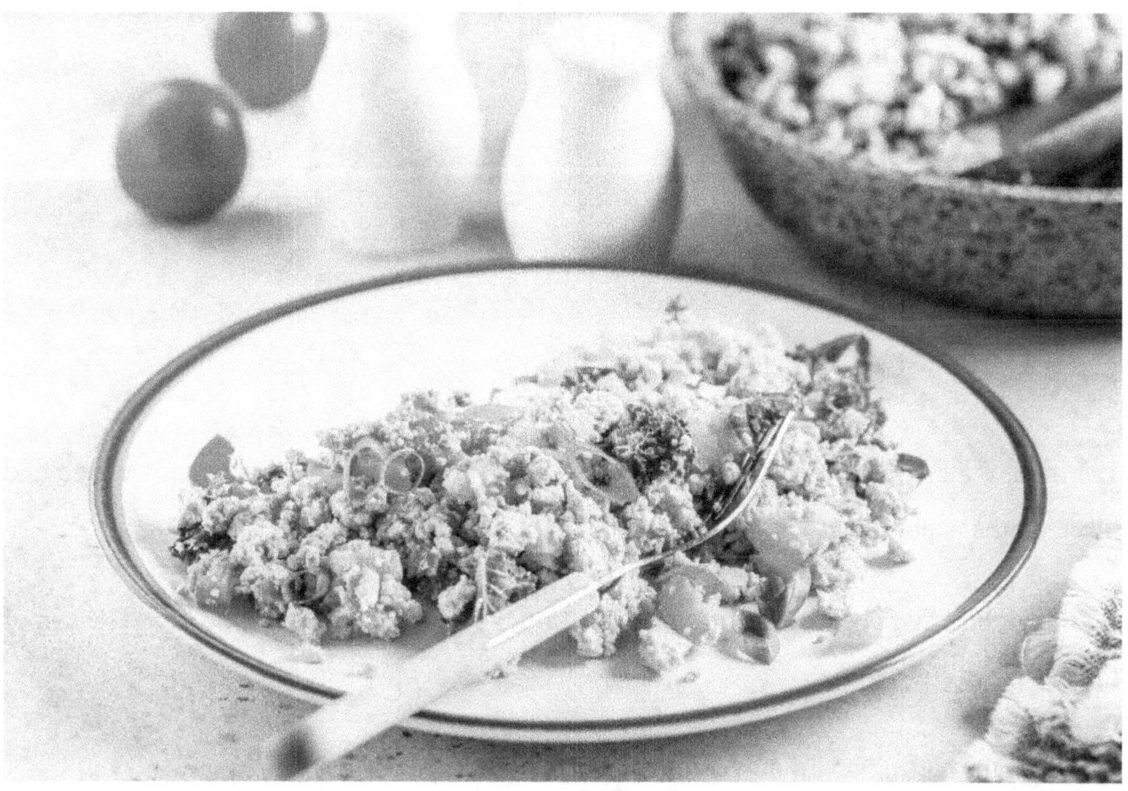

Scrambled tofu is the perfect source of nutrition as it is packed with a range of nutrients that will suit your bodily needs. It takes a shorter time to prepare.

Servings: 4

Cook time: 40 minutes

Ingredients:

- ¼ tsp. onion powder
- 1 c. cherry tomatoes, quartered
- 14 oz. extra-firm tofu
- 1 tsp. ground turmeric
- 1 tsp. olive oil
- ¼ tsp. garlic powder

Directions:

1. Line a plate with several paper towels. Remove the tofu block from the package and place on the paper towels.

2. Add additional paper towels on top of the tofu block and place a cutting board on top of the paper towels.

3. Weigh the cutting board down with a heavy book, a pot, or several cans.

4. Leave the tofu to drain for at least 30 minutes.

5. In a large sauté pan or skillet, heat the olive oil on medium heat and add the block of tofu.

6. Mash the tofu into small curds with a potato masher.

7. Stir in the turmeric, onion powder, garlic powder, and tomatoes and sauté together for 5 minutes.

8. Serve.

Rainbow chard and sweet potato hash

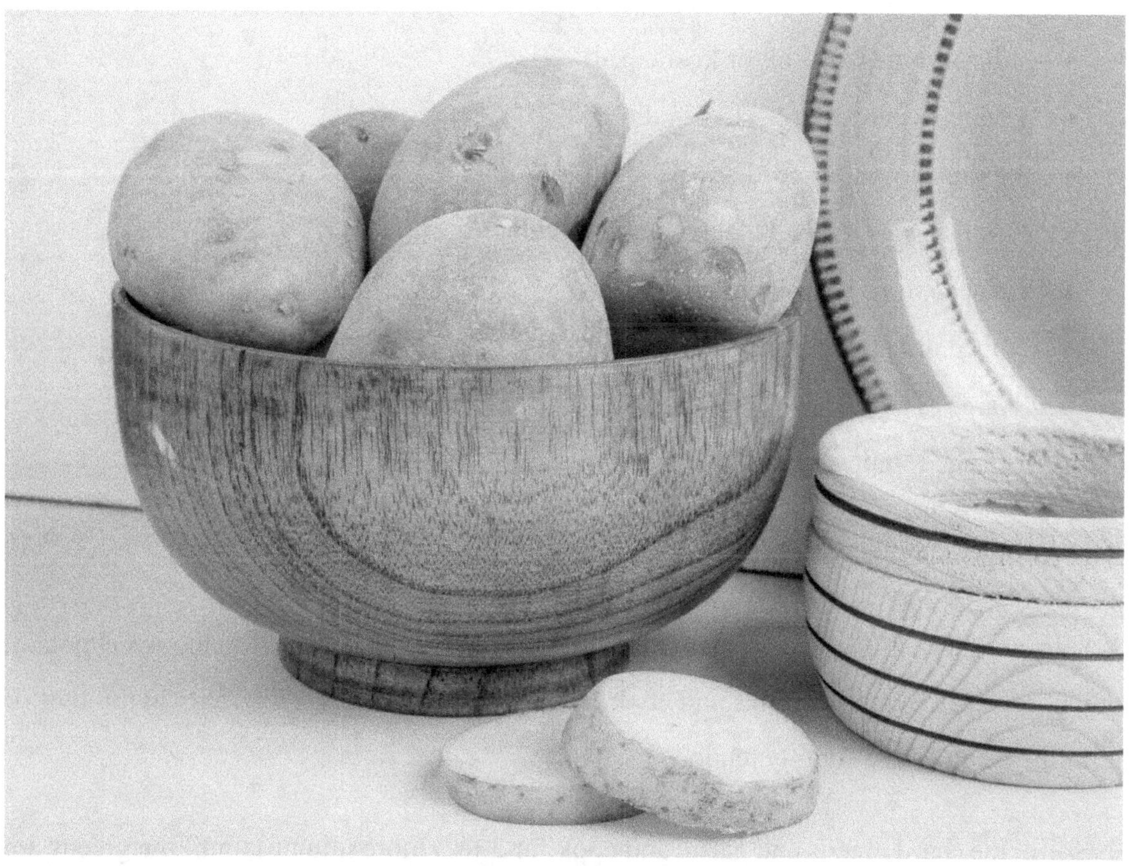

If you need a delicacy that is packed with nutrition, then Rainbow chard and sweet potato hash is a perfect option. You will enjoy!

Servings: 3

Cook time: 30 minutes

Ingredients:

- ¼ tsp. red pepper flakes, crushed
- ¾ tsp. divided sea salt or kosher salt
- 1 large sweet potato, skin-on, diced
- 3 garlic cloves, minced
- ½ tsp. freshly ground black pepper, divided
- 3 tbsp. extra-virgin olive oil
- ¼ medium sweet onion, diced
- 8 large eggs
- 1 bunch rainbow chard, chopped

Directions:

1. Set a nonstick skillet over medium high heat. Add olive oil to heat. Add the sweet potato, onion, and rainbow chard stalks and cook, as you stir occasionally, for 15 to 20 minutes or until the potatoes are slightly tender.

2. Stir in the chard greens and garlic and cook for 2 to 3 more minutes, until the greens are wilted. Stir in ½ teaspoon of the salt, ¼ teaspoon of the black pepper, and the pepper flakes.

3. Use a spatula to create eight wells in the hash. Crack an egg into each well, season with the remaining ¼ teaspoon salt and ¼ teaspoon black pepper and place a lid on the skillet. Cook for 4 to 5 more minutes, until the egg whites are cooked through.

4. Store the hash in a microwaveable airtight container and refrigerate for up to 5 days. Reheat it by microwaving on high for 1 to 3 minutes, until heated through.

Vegetable-Avocado Toast

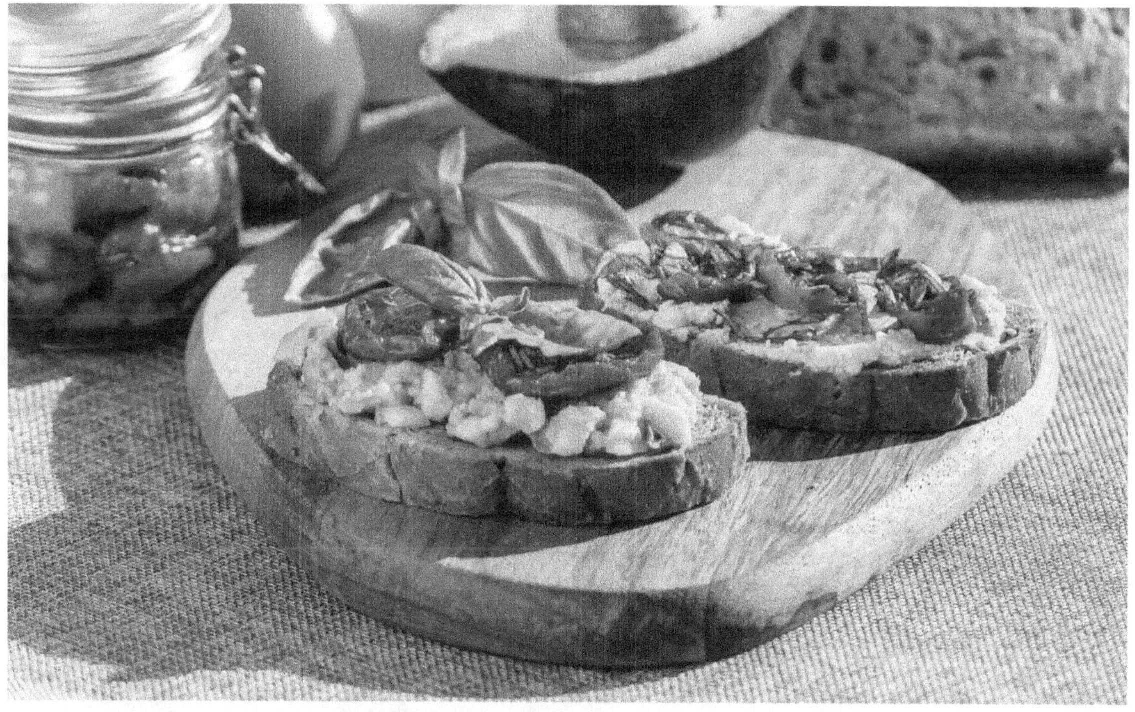

The Vegetable-Avocado toast is prepared using a few essential ingredients such as arugula, olive oil, whole grain bread, among others. The avocado can serve as a substitute for butter for the toast. Enjoy your morning nutritiously by preparing this meal.

Servings: 4

Cook time: 5 minutes

Ingredients:

- 1 c. fresh arugula
- 1 tsp. cracked black pepper
- 1 large avocado
- 4 pieces of whole-grain bread
- 1 beet, peeled
- 2 tbsp. olive oil

Directions:

1. Remove the pit, peel the avocado, and cut into 4 portions, set aside.

2. Shave the beet on a box grater; set aside.

3. Toast the bread to your liking.

4. Top the toast with the avocado, arugula, and shaved beets.

5. Drizzle the toast with olive oil, sprinkle with cracked pepper, and serve.

Scrambles

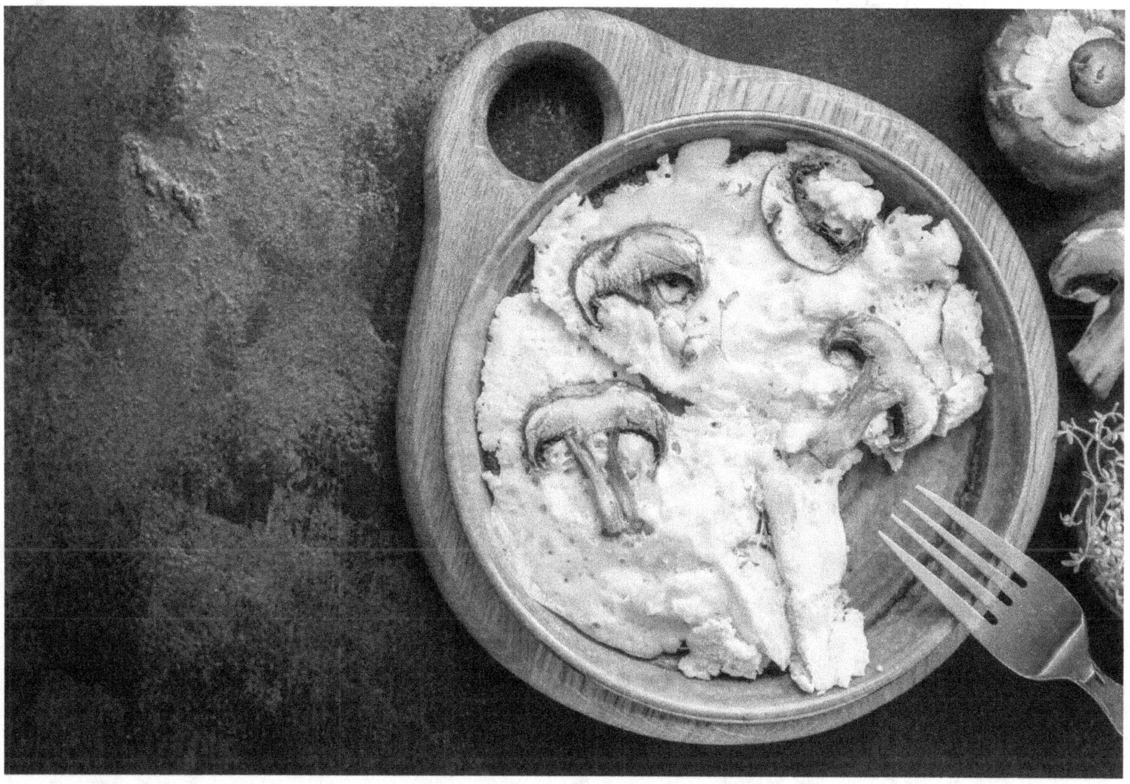

You will only need scrambled eggs, mushroom, onion, olive oil, and spinach. A combination of veggies and eggs will work well for you. It is an excellent way of preparing a breakfast that will keep you strengthened all through the day.

Servings: 2

Cook time: 25 minutes

Ingredients:

- 2 eggs, scrambled.
- ¼ c. sliced mushrooms.
- ¼ c. chopped onions.
- Olive oil.
- ½ c. young spinach.

Directions:

1. Using a pan, add enough olive oil to prevent vegetables from sticking.

2. Add in mushrooms and onions, set heat to low and fry as you stir until onions become translucent and mushrooms just start to turn green.

3. Add in the spinach, stir before just beginning to wilt. Remove eggs and whisk to mix.

4. Scrape the mixture as they begin to cook. Flip the mixture when the eggs are almost done.

5. Cook to desired moistness/dryness.

Frittata

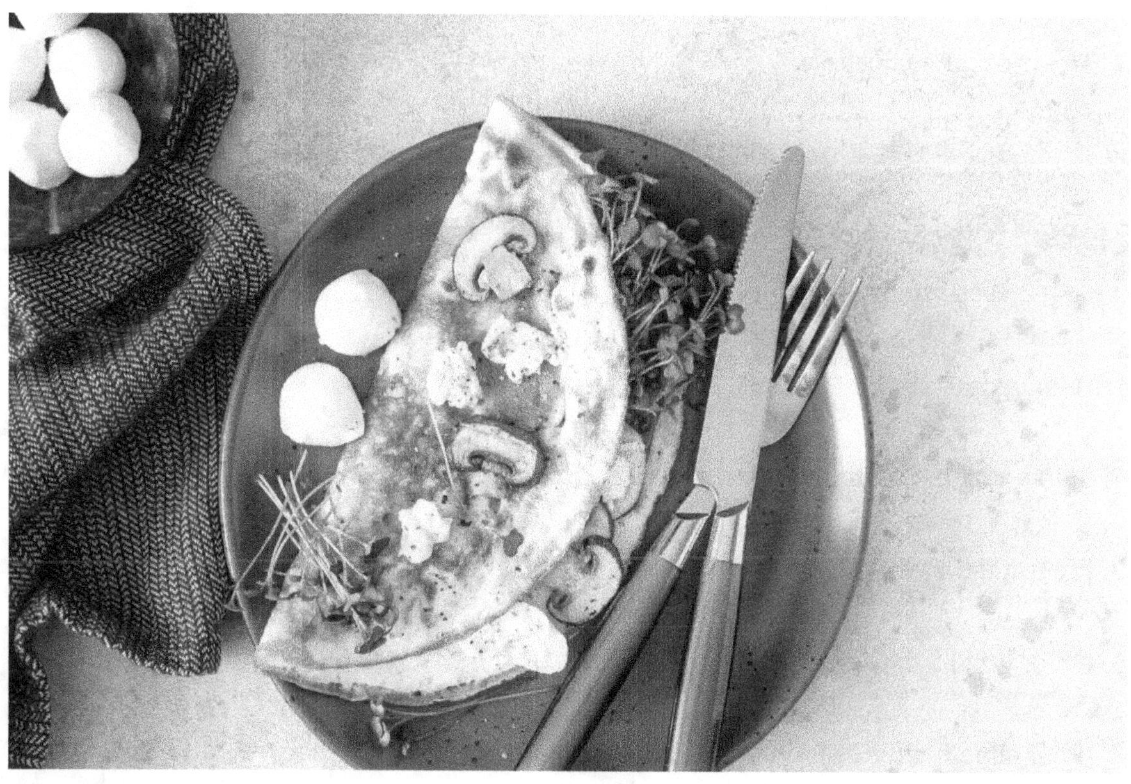

The weekend mornings can always be better with a nicely prepared frittata. The goodness with it is versatility. The ingredients are easily accessible, and the entire preparation process is easier.

Servings: 3

Cook time: 20 minutes

Ingredients:

- ¼ c. sliced mushrooms.
- 1 oz. grated cheese.
- Olive oil
- ¼ c. chopped onions.
- ½ c. young spinach.
- 3 eggs scrambled.

Directions:

1. Start with one egg in the same way as the scramble:

2. Preheat the oven to 350 ° F.

3. Oil or grind 3 cups of muffin or cupcakes

4. Pour ample olive oil into the pot to avoid sticking vegetables. Add onions and mushrooms, fry over low heat, and stir until the onions are slightly translucent and mushrooms begin to change color. Apply spinach, stir until it wakes. Connect the eggs and blend.

5. Put into the three muffin tins and divided evenly.

6. Sprinkle the cheese, split evenly.

7. Bake for 15 to 20 minutes, slightly melted eggs and cheese.

Omelet

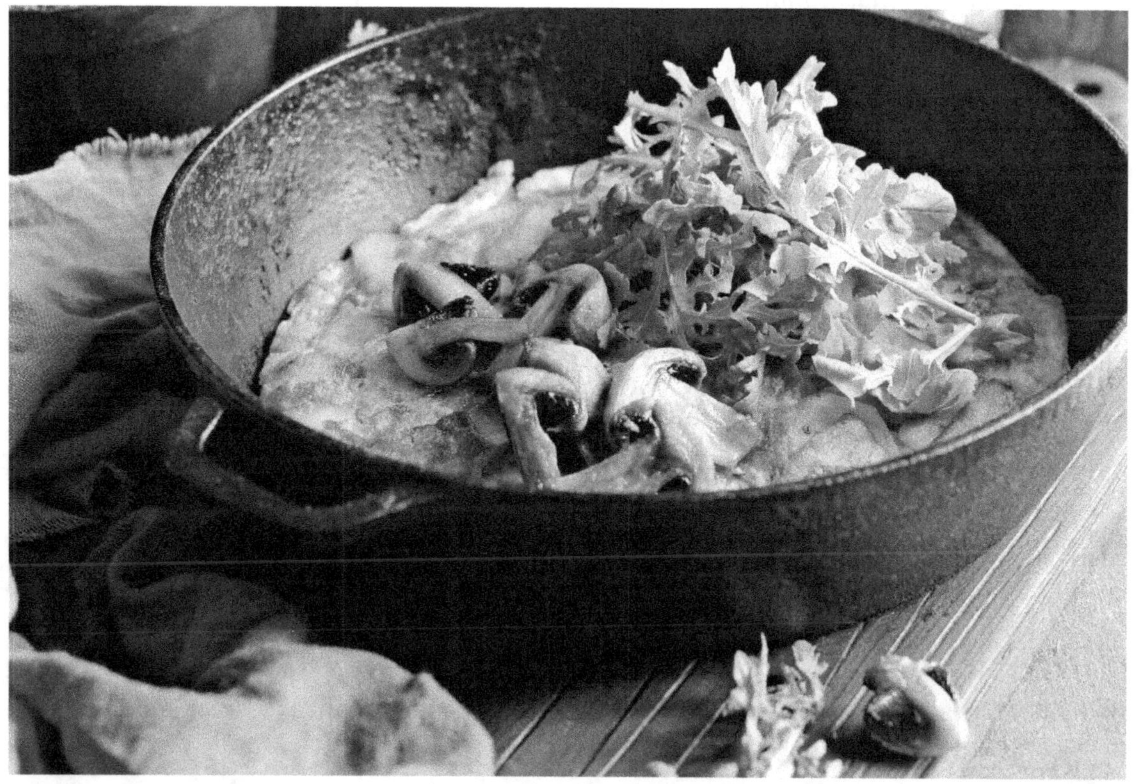

If your morning is kind of busy, you have to choose a meal that is easy to prepare with affordable and easily accessible ingredients. When nicely prepared, a combination of olive oil, onions, spinach, eggs, and mushroom is enough to produce a delicious omelet. Enjoy it.

Servings: 2

Cook time: 10 minutes

Ingredients:

- ¼ c. sliced mushrooms.
- 2 eggs scrambled.
- ½ c. young spinach.
- ¼ c. chopped onions.
- Olive oil.
- 2 tbsp. Grated cheese

Directions:

1. In a little olive oil, cook the vegetables. Hold warm on low heat.

2. Place the eggs in a bowl or omelet.

3. Cook over low heat until the eggs are set in the pancake shape. Flip and cook until the eggs are done a little longer. Pile the veggies on top, fold the "pancake" over and inside the veggies.

4. Apply 2 tablespoons grated cheese before folding the pancakes or sprinkle the 2 tablespoons on top of the omelet if you prefer cheese in the omelet.

Easy Gluten-Free Berry Crisp

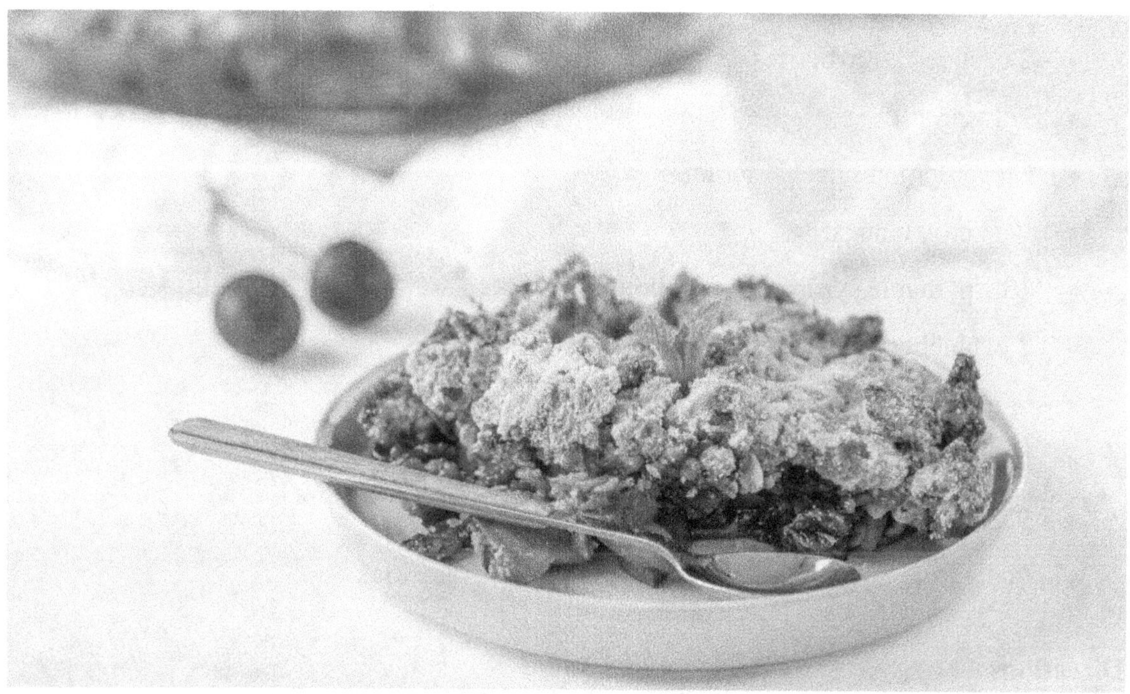

A blend of eleven nutritious ingredients would serve better for any member of the family. The meal is rich in ingredients that will give you a perfect starter for the day.

Servings: 3

Cook time: 20 minutes

Ingredients:

- 2 tbsp. chia seeds.
- 2 c. sliced strawberries.
- 1/8 tsp. salt.
- Meyer lemon juice, ½ lemon
- ¼ c. brown sugar.
- 1 tbsp. maple syrup optional though.
- 2 c. blueberries.
- ½ c. gluten-free oats.
- ¼ c. tapioca starch.
- ¼ c. brown rice flour.
- ¼ c. virgin coconut oil melted, plus extra for ramekins.

Directions:

1. Preheat oven to 350 ° F. In a mixing bowl, add strawberries, blueberries, lemon juice, and chia seeds.

2. Add oats, flour, brown sugar, coconut oil, and salt together in another cup.

3. Grease 4 ramekins with coconut oil, then spoon fruit mix into ramekins and combine oatmeal/flour. Place about 20 minutes on a baking sheet or until it is crispy.

4. Remove slightly from the oven to cool, then serve.

Banana-Nut Breakfast Porridge

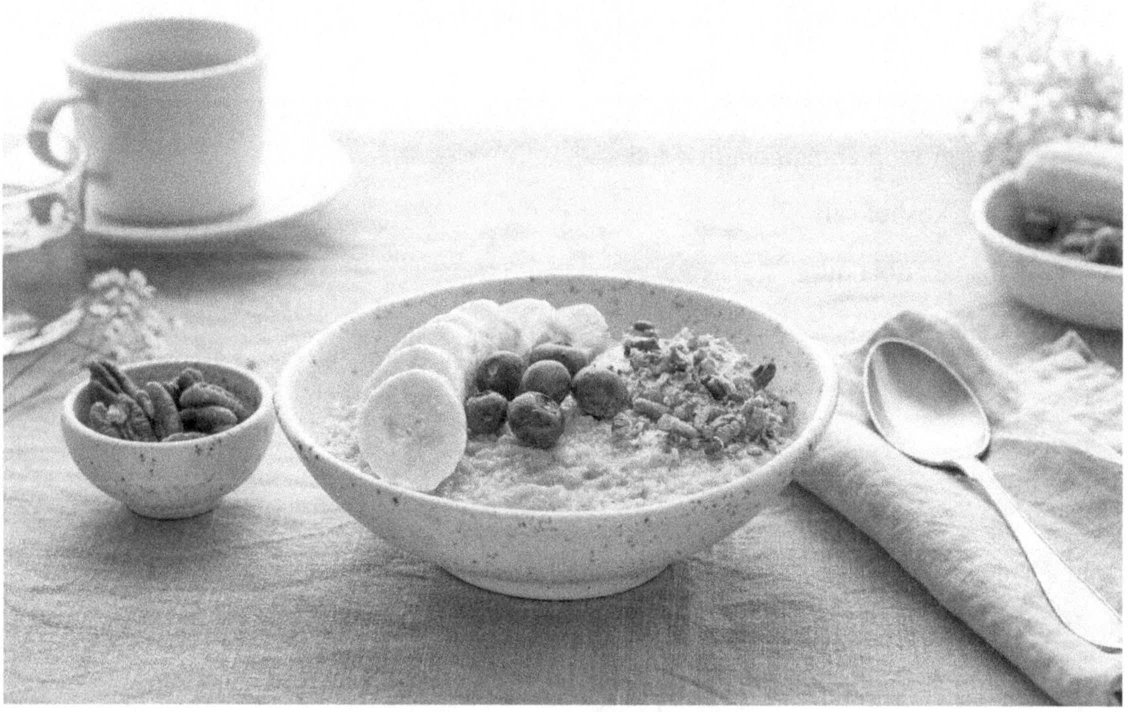

Perhaps there is not a better way to start your chilly morning other than the Banana-nut Breakfast porridge. The meal is loaded with ingredients that will perfectly boost your entire body health.

Servings: 8

Cook time: 40 minutes

Ingredients:

- 2 medium bananas, peeled and sliced
- ½ c. chopped unsalted almonds
- ¼ c. packed brown sugar
- ½ tsp. pure vanilla extract
- 1 tsp. ground cinnamon, divided
- ¼ tsp. kosher salt
- 1 tbsp. canola oil
- 2 c. farro
- 5 c. milk

Directions:

1. In a saucepan over medium heat, bring the farro and milk to a low simmer. Cook for 25 to 30 minutes, stirring frequently, until the farro is soft and most of the liquid has been absorbed. Stir in the brown sugar, vanilla, salt, and ½ teaspoon of the cinnamon.

2. Heat a dry skillet over medium-low heat. Add the almonds and toast, stirring constantly, for 30 to 60 seconds or until they are lightly browned. Remove the nuts from the skillet and set them aside.

3. Return the skillet to the stove over medium heat and add the oil. When the oil is hot, add the sliced bananas, sprinkle them with the remaining ½ teaspoon of cinnamon, and sauté for 1 to 2 minutes per side, until the bananas are browned and caramelized.

4. Serve the porridge with the caramelized bananas and toasted nuts.

5. Store the porridge in a microwaveable airtight container and refrigerate for up to 4 days. Serve it cold or reheat it by microwaving on high for 1 to 3 minutes until heated through.

Main Dishes

Since the main dishes are the most essential in your diet, we have picked out the best of all other meals to serve as the essential providers of desired nutrients. Most of the meals here are rich in nutrients that help expand and grow the health of your brain. You can enjoy them with friends and family members.

Salmon-Kale Summer Rolls

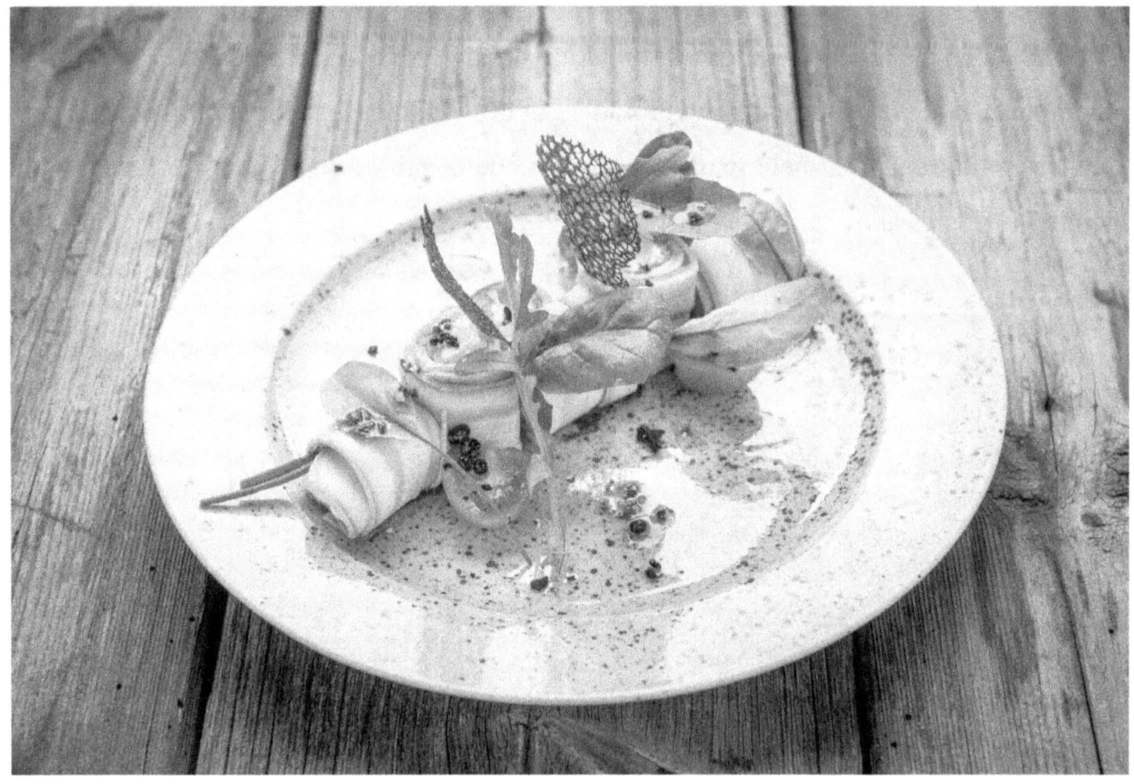

A new way of boosting your day's mood is to try the salmon-kale summer rolls. It entails a range of ingredients that are good for your health. Enjoy the Salmon-Kale Summer rolls.

Servings: 4

Cook time: 55 minutes

Ingredients:

- 1 tbsp. canola oil.
- 2 tsp. light brown sugar.
- 1 ½ c. very thinly sliced English cucumbers
- 6 oz. thinly sliced smoked salmon.
- 4 ½ tbsp. rice vinegar, divided.
- ¾ tsp. kosher salt, divided.
- 5 large Lacinato kale leaves stems removed.
- 8 round rice paper sheets.
- 1 ½ very thinly sliced radishes
- 1 sliced avocado, 16 slices.

Directions:

1. In a strainer, put rice. Rinse under cold running water for about 1 minute until clear.

2. Move rice to a tiny cup, add 1 ½ cups of water. Cover and put over high heat to a boil.

3. Reduce to medium-low heat and cook 40 minutes. Remove from heat and allow 20 minutes to stand.

4. Transfer to a medium-sized bowl and toss with sugar, 3 ½ vinegar tablespoon, and 1⁄2 salt teaspoon. Let it cool about 20 minutes.

5. Put kale in a bowl with olive oil and one tablespoon of vinegar and 1⁄4 teaspoon of salt. Massage vigorously with fingers for 1 to 2 minutes, until the leaves are tender.

6. Fill a large, shallow dish with warm water at a depth of 1 inch. Place one sheet of rice on the water; let stand only about 30 seconds until soft. Move to a smooth surface of the sheet.

7. Arrange 1/8 of the radishes, 1/8 of the cucumbers, and two avocado pieces in a row across the wrapper center, leaving at every end a 1-inch margin. Finish with 1⁄4 cup of rice, pinch together grains as you seal.

8. Add 1⁄4 cup of peanut and 3⁄4 ounce of salmon. Fold the ends of the sheet and roll up, jelly-roll mode. Push the seam gently to close.

9. Place roll, seam side down, on a platter lined in a damp towel or paper, and cover with another damp towel of paper so that it is not dry.

10. Repeat the rest of the ingredients cycle. Serve immediately.

Greek Style Chicken Wraps

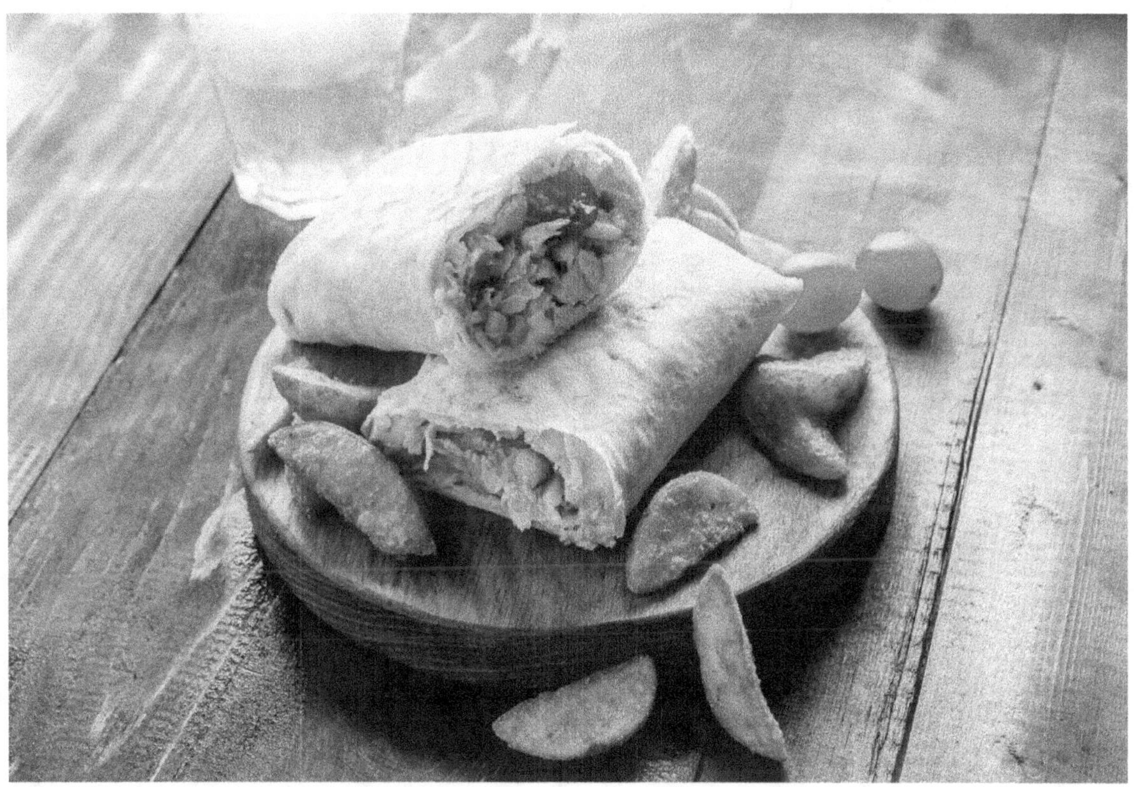

The chicken wraps are just a go-to meal when you are in dire need of a sweet option of wraps. The recipe is loaded with a range of unique ingredients that serves as a perfect choice for anyone who needs to grow health-wise.

Servings: 6

Cook time: 1 minute

Ingredients:

- 1 c. shredded boneless, skinless rotisserie chicken breast
- 1 c. halved grape tomatoes
- 6 pieces 8-inch whole-wheat flour tortillas
- 1 tbsp. chopped fresh oregano
- 1/8 tsp. ground red pepper
- 3 tbsp. coarsely chopped pitted Kalamata olives
- 1 ½ tbsp. fresh lemon juice
- 1 tbsp. olive oil
- 2 small or Kirby cucumbers, chopped
- 6 tbsp. plain hummus

Directions:

1. Toss feta, chicken, cucumber, pepper, oregano, olives, tomatoes, oil and juice in a large mixing bowl.

2. Scoop 1 tablespoon of hummus over each tortilla. Spread all over. Scoop ½ cup of chicken mixture over one side of the tortilla's surface.

3. Carefully roll the tortilla and slice each wrap in half. Serve.

Dreamy Turkey and Veggie English Muffin Sammie

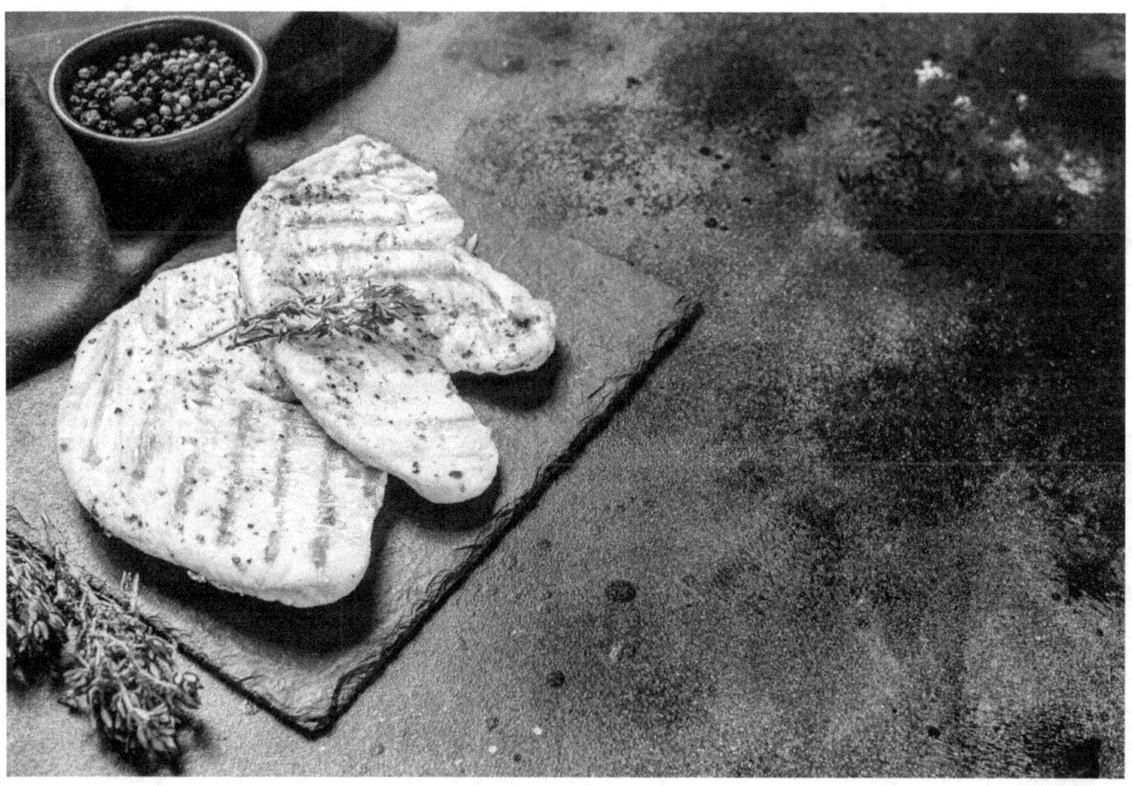

The excellent Sammie entails ingredients such as Romaine lettuce leaf, salt and pepper, some slices of radish and some ripe avocado, among other ingredients. The meal is a perfect option to prepare you for the day. Enjoy it.

Servings: 2

Cook time: 2 minutes

Ingredients:

- 1 halved English muffin, whole-grain and toasted.
- ½ Romaine lettuce leaf.
- ¼ ripe avocado.
- 3 oz. roasted turkey breast, sliced.
- Fresh squeezed juice, ½ lime.
- Salt and ground pepper to taste.
- 1 sliced radish

Directions:

1. Place your English muffin in a toaster. Toast for about 60 seconds, depending on how you like it toasted. Remove the plate and set aside.

2. Spread a pinch of salt and pepper and sprinkle on half of your muffin together with the avocado, spray with the lime juice. Cover with slices of radish.

3. Pile up the breast of turkey and lettuce. To complete the sandwich, top with the other remaining half on top.

Easy Lentil Salad with Lemon Vinaigrette

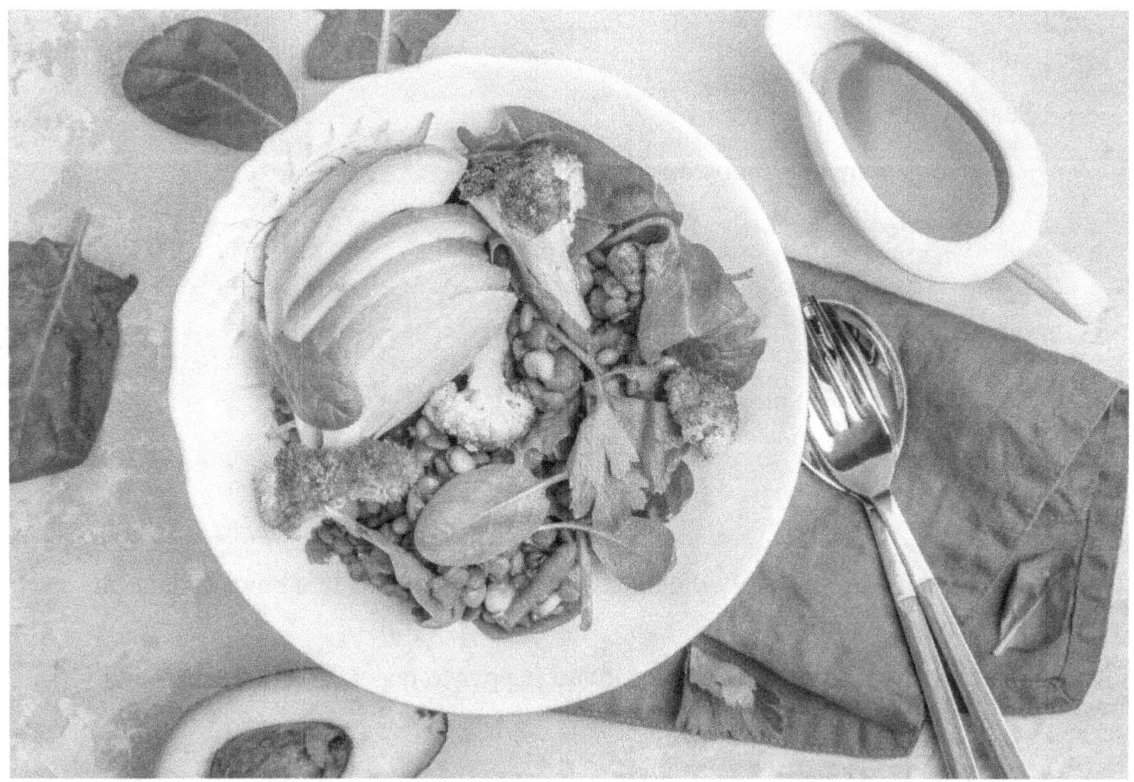

You can get the perfect outcome from the Lentil salad by incorporating some lemony taste. It is excellent to try it along with lemon vinaigrette. You can enjoy the natural flavors along with your friends.

Servings: 2

Cook time: 3 minutes

Ingredients:

- 1 tbsp. extra-virgin olive oil.
- 2 c. chopped kale.
- Sea salt and black pepper
- ¾ c. cherry tomatoes, halved.
- ½ c. chopped Radicchio.
- 2 tbsp. slivered almonds.
- ½ c. cooked lentils.
- Lemon juice, ¼ lemon.

Directions:

1. Place kale, cherry tomatoes, Radicchio, lentils, and almonds in a bowl of salads.

2. Add olive oil, citrus fruit juice, and salt and pepper to taste. Then toss thoroughly, then serve.

Salmon Superfood Noodle Bowl

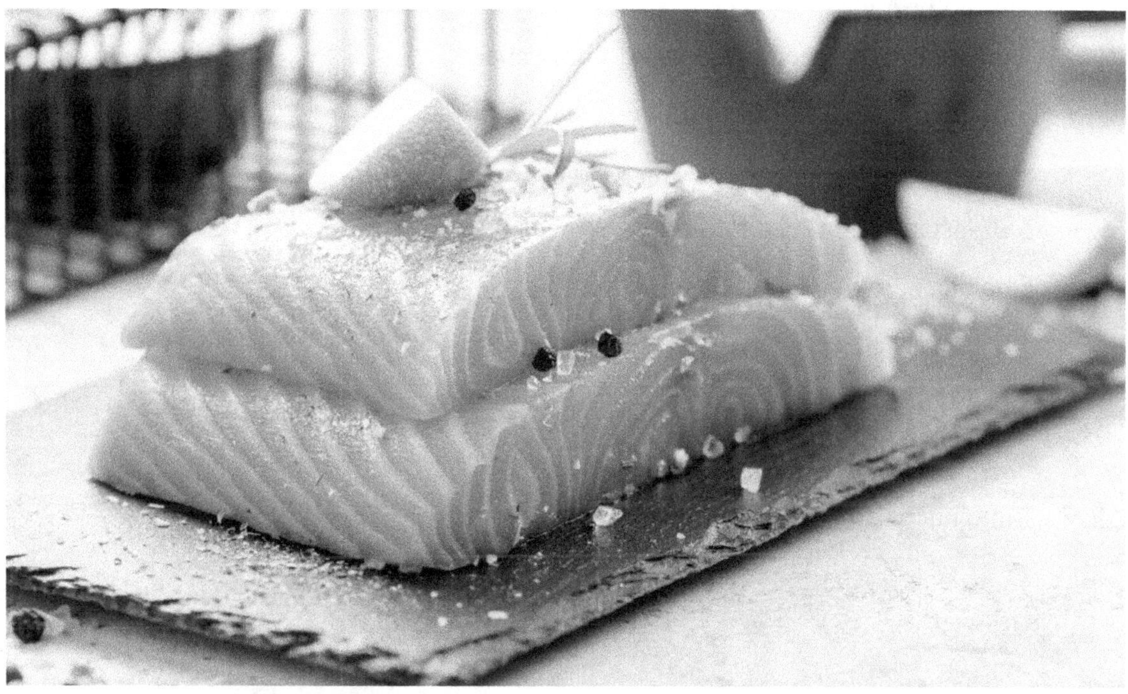

The sweetness from a meal you will always love comes from the Salmon superfood noodle bowl. Don't miss out on the added sweet salmon taste.

Servings: 2

Cook time: 20 minutes

Ingredients:

- ¼ tsp. black pepper
- 4 oz. cucumber, keep the skin on, thinly sliced
- ½ small avocado, sliced into bite-size pieces
- 1 6-oz. salmon fillet, skinless, 8 pieces
- 5 oz. asparagus, sliced into thirds
- Cooking spray
- 1 tbsp. toasted sesame oil
- ¼ tsp. salt
- 4 oz. whole-wheat spaghetti or soba buckwheat noodles
- Lime juice and zest, 2 limes

Directions:

1. Boil some water in a deep pot and cook the noodles until al dente. The noodles should cook for around 6 minutes while spaghetti cooks for about 8 minutes. Once noodles are done, strain them and set aside. Reserve the pasta water.

2. In the same water where you cooked the pasta, put asparagus. Cook for about 2 minutes until it turns bright green and al dente.

3. Drain and rinse the asparagus under cold running water. Place a skillet or grill pan over a stove set to medium high heat. Spray cooking oil over the skillet or grill pan to grease it lightly.

4. Once the skillet or pan is hot, place the salmon pieces. Cook salmon until done, about 2 to 3 minutes on each side. Transfer cooked salmon on a plate and set aside.

5. Pour lime juice and sesame oil into a small bowl. Add lime zest and season with pepper and salt. Whisk together to create vinaigrette.

6. Place the noodles in a medium-sized serving plate. Add asparagus, avocados and cucumbers. Pour the vinaigrette all over. Toss to combine.

7. Top with salmon and serve.

Seared Chicken Thigh with Pepper & Celery Caponata

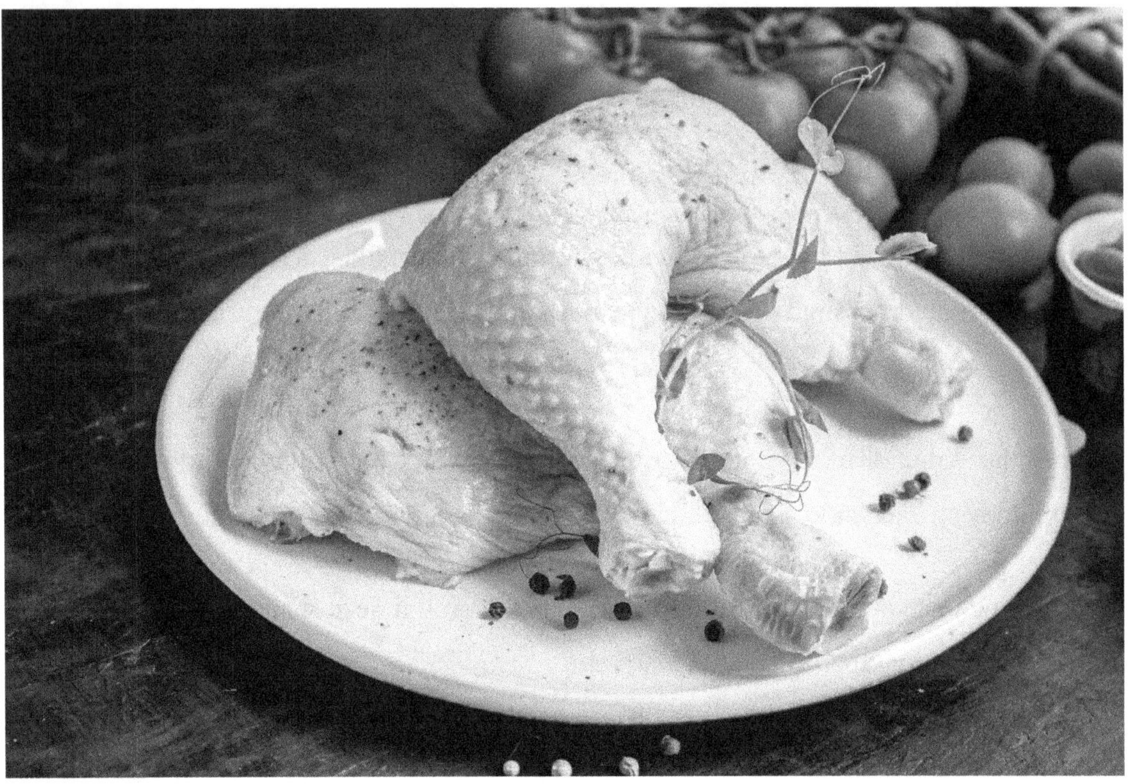

Chicken will always be sweet when incorporated with a few essential ingredients and toppings. Enjoy some added hotness from the pepper.

Servings: 4

Cook time: 41 minutes

Ingredients:

- 200 g chicken thigh
- 140 g fresh spinach

For the caponata:

- Oil spray
- 1 red onion, sliced
- ½ tsp. dried oregano
- 1 (400-g) can chopped tomato
- 1 orange pepper, deseeded, sliced into quarters
- 1 tbsp. caper
- 2 garlic cloves, sliced into slivers
- 25g black pitted Kalamata olive, sliced in half
- 2 sticks of celery, sliced crosswise
- 1 tsp. balsamic vinegar

Directions:

1. Lightly coat a wide, large non-stick skillet with cooking spray. Place over a stove set to medium high heat. Put the garlic and onions. Cover the skillet and cook the garlic and onions for 5 minutes. Stir halfway to brown them evenly.

2. Put the tomatoes into the skillet. Fill the can of the tomatoes with water and pour into the skillet as well.

3. Stir and place the rest of the ingredients for the caponata. Cover and let the caponata simmer on low heat setting for 30 minutes. Take a small frying pan or griddle, heat over a stove set to high.

4. Sprinkle a generous amount of ground black pepper all over the chicken. Sear the chicken on both sides. This will take about 8 minutes to sear both sides or until no longer pink inside.

5. Set another pan over low heat. Place the spinach and cover. Cook until the spinach leaves are wilted. Transfer to a plate.

6. Divide the caponata between 2 serving plates. Arrange the spinach on top. Slice the chicken into strips and arrange them on top of the spinach.

7. Serve immediately.

Superfood Salmon Burgers

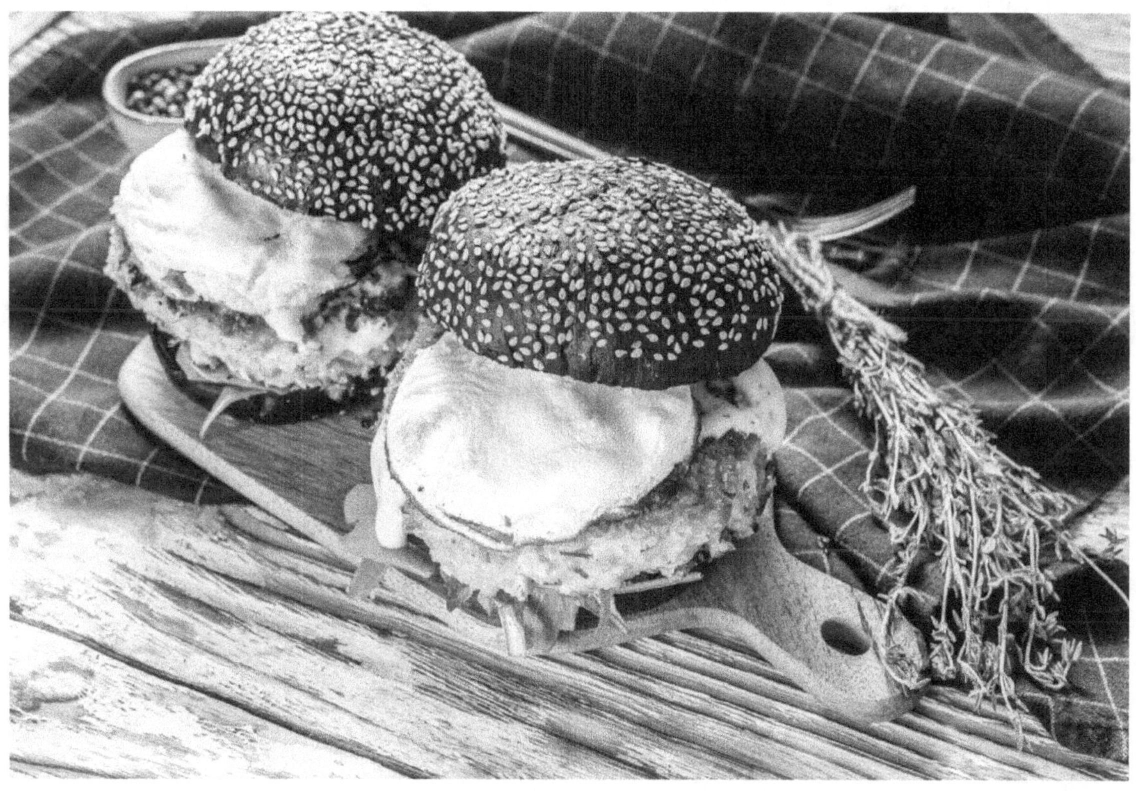

At times you will always need something lighter and delicious. With an easy way of preparation, Superfood salmon burgers will give you that perfect taste of salmon in a burger. Enjoy the meal with friends and family.

Servings: 4

Cook time: 10 minutes

Ingredients:

- 1 tsp. soy sauce
- 4 skinless, boneless salmon fillets, slice into medium-sized chunks
- Lemon, sliced into wedges
- Thumb-size fresh piece ginger root, grated
- 1 tsp. vegetable oil
- 1 bunch coriander, picked leaves from half of the bunch, chop the other
- 2 tbsp. Thai red curry paste

For the salad:

- 2 tbsp. white wine vinegar
- 1 tsp. golden caster sugar
- 2 medium-sized carrots

Directions:

1. Put salmon in a food processor.

2. Add soy, chopped coriander, ginger and paste. Pulse the mixture until ingredients are roughly minced. Transfer into a shallow dish.

3. Divide the mixture into 4. Form each portion into burger patties.

4. Heat oil in a frying pan set over high heat. Once oil and pan are hot, fry burgers for about 4 to 5 minutes a side. Slice cucumber and carrots into thin strips using a swivel peeler.

5. Add sugar and vinegar to the vegetables strips. Mix until all the sugar dissolves. Add coriander leaves and toss.

6. Put salad on a plate, divided between 4 serving plates.

7. Place a small serving of rice on each plate and top with one burger.

Salmon with Broad Bean Salad

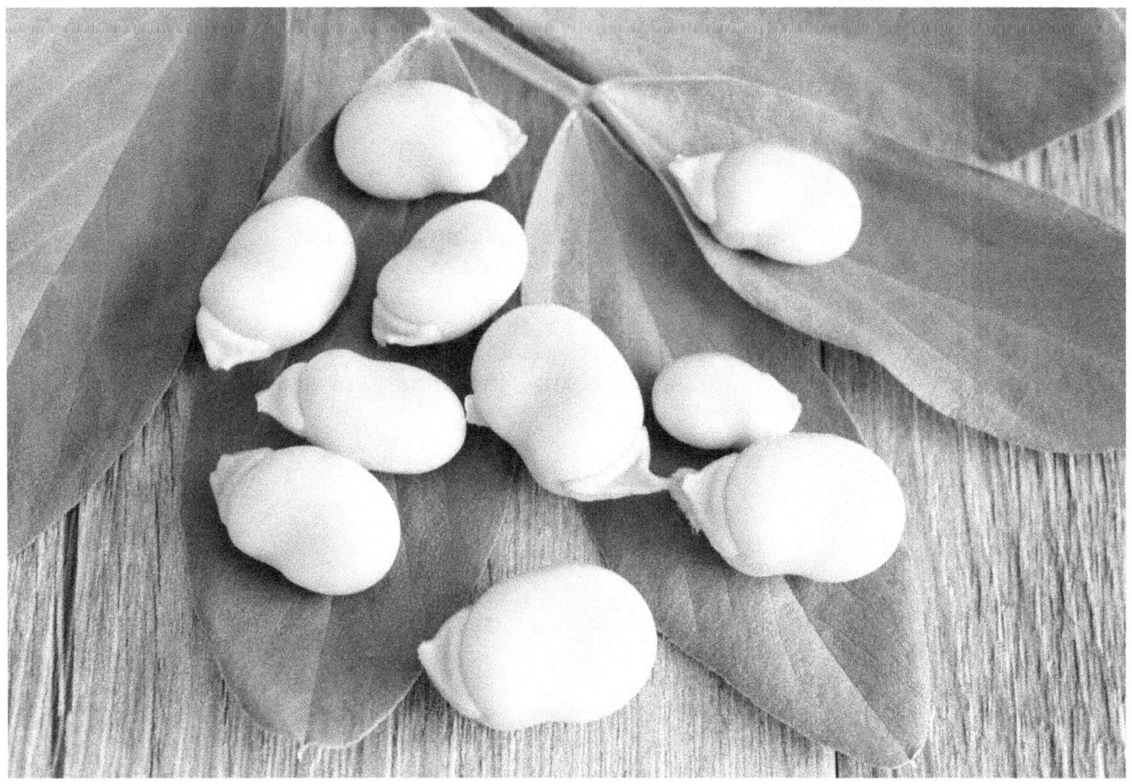

A salad of broad bean and the taste of seafood such as salmon works much better when added toppings and stuffing are incorporated. Within a short period, your meal will be ready.

Servings: 4

Cook time: 16 minutes

Ingredients:

- 1 lemon, sliced into wedges
- 200 g tub roasted artichoke hearts in oil, drain but reserve its oil
- 2 raw lightly smoked salmon fillets
- 4 spring onions, trimmed and sliced
- 250 g broad beans, fresh or frozen, removed from the pods
- 300 g small new potatoes, sliced in half
- Black pepper, freshly ground
- 3 tbsp. extra virgin olive oil
- Lemon zest, 2 preserved small lemons
- Salt
- Handful of fresh mint leaves, sliced
- 100 g wild rocket

Directions:

1. Boil water in a large pot and cook the potatoes for 10 minutes, or until fork tender.

2. Put the beans into this same pot. Cook until just tender. Drain the vegetables. Rinse with running cold water to stop further cooking.

3. Put potatoes in a large bowl. Pour in the oil reserved from the artichokes.

4. Stir to coat the potatoes.

5. Add more olive oil as necessary. Set aside to continue cooling. Once cooled, place potatoes in a serving plate. Remove the skins from the beans and place in a bowl.

6. Place artichokes pieces into the bowl with the beans. Put in sliced preserved lemons, remaining olive oil, seasoning and spring onions. Toss to mix.

7. Place a small pan on a stove set to medium high heat.

8. Once pan is hot, cook the fish, skin-side down first. Cook for 3 minutes then flip to cook the other side.

9. Lower the heat and cover the pan to finish cooking the fish. Turn the heat off. Let the fish cool slightly before handling. Remove the skin from the fish. Flake the fish and remove any bones. Add into the bowl with the beans. Add rocket and mint. Toss and spoon over the potatoes. Serve with some lemon.

Chicken and Wheat Berry Bowl

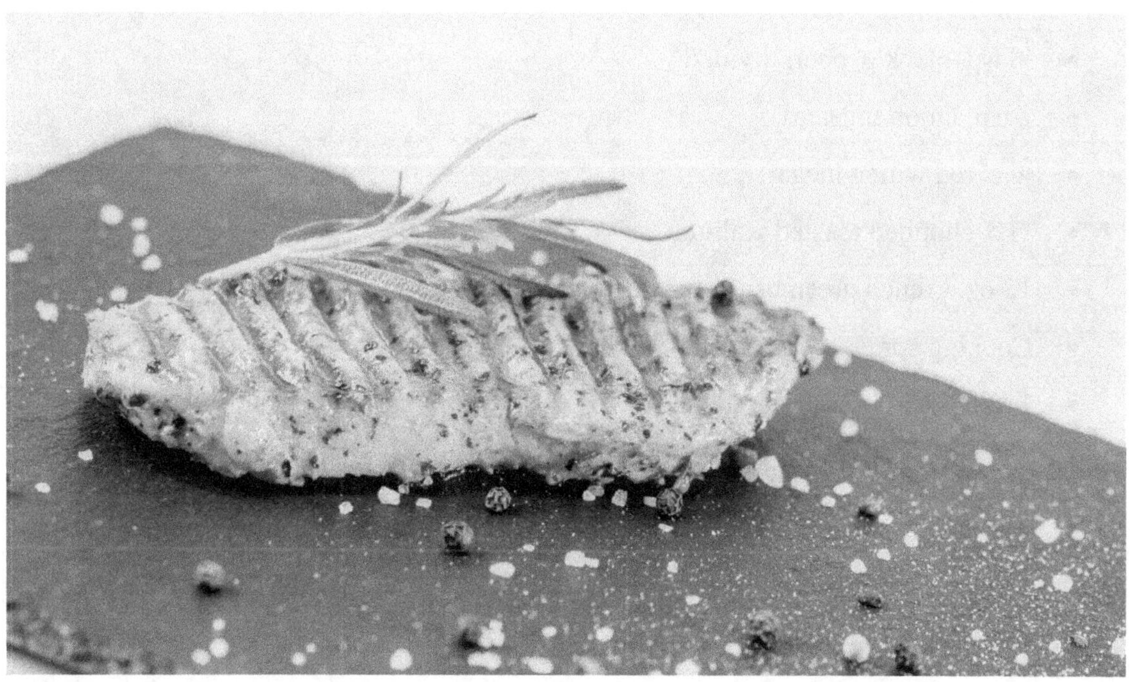

The incorporation of some brain-boosting grains into a specially prepared chicken sounds fantastic. It is delicious and nutritious.

Servings: 3

Cook time: 1 hour

Ingredients:

- ¾ c. uncooked hard wheat berries
- ½ tsp. black pepper, divided.
- 2 tsp. Dijon mustard.
- ¼ c. red wine vinegar.
- ½ c. chopped toasted walnuts.
- 12 oz. French green beans trimmed and cut into 2-inch pieces.
- Cooking spray.
- 1 ¼ tsp. kosher salt, divided.
- ¼ c. olive oil.
- 1 ½ tbsp. chopped fresh tarragon.
- 2 boneless, skinless chicken breasts.
- 2 c. fresh blueberries

Directions:

1. Hold a large pot of boiling water. Remove the wheat berries, reduce the heat to medium and cook for 45 to 50 minutes until tender.

2. Stir in green beans and cook for 3 minutes. Drain the wheat and beans and rinse them with cold water until they are fresh. Transfer to a bowl. Transfer.

3. Cover a spray cast iron barbecue pot or skillet and heat to medium-high. Sprinkle the chicken with ½ salt teaspoon and ¼ pepper teaspoon. Add the chicken and grill to 160 ° F, approximately 5 minutes per side.

4. Transfer the chicken to a cutting board and leave for 5 minutes to rest before cutting.

5. Meanwhile, whisk the remaining ¾ teaspoon salt, vinegar, tarragon, mouth, and ¼ teaspoon pepper together.

6. In a bowl, add the blueberries, walnuts, and vinaigrette to the wheat berry mixture.

7. Split the mixture evenly between 4 shallow bowls.

8. Slice the chicken into the grain, then break the chicken into bowls.

Tuna and Avocado Egg Salad

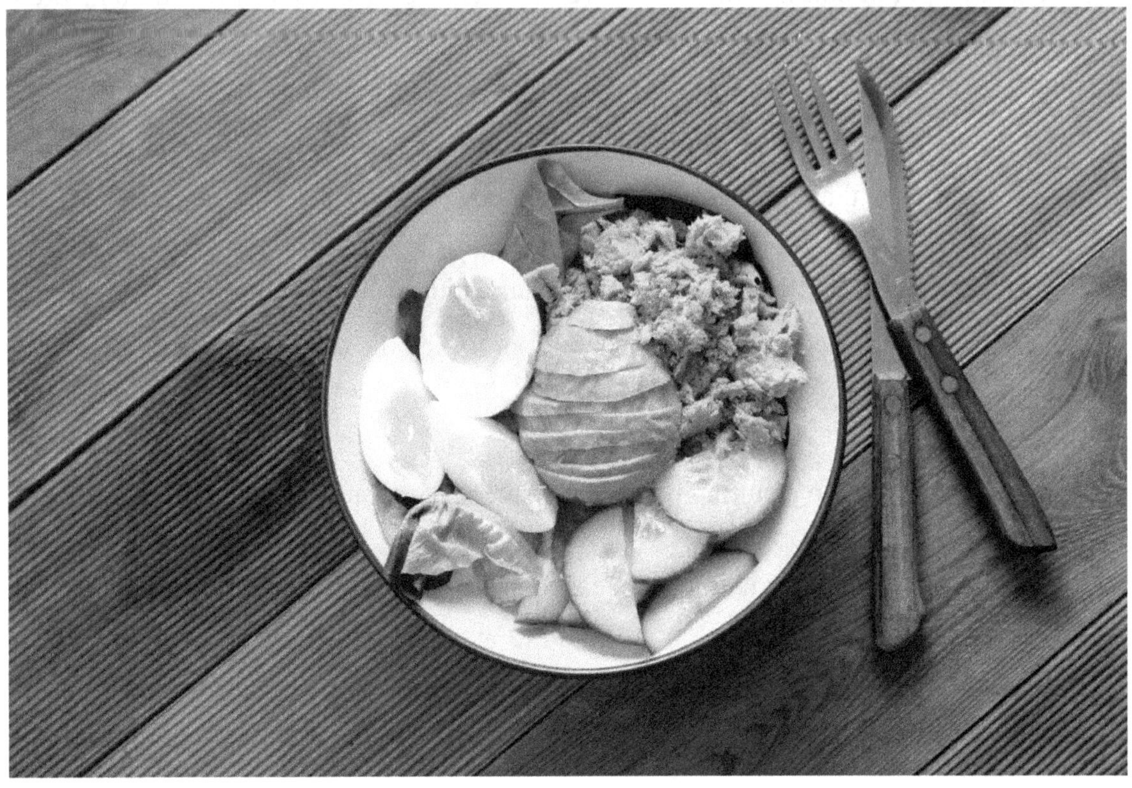

Tuna and Avocado Egg salad can be easily prepared just in a few minutes. The meal is a perfect alternative to any nutritious salad. Enjoy it.

Servings: 6

Cook time: 18 minutes

Ingredients:

- 1 tbsp. mayonnaise
- Lemon juice, ½ medium lemon
- ¼ tsp. freshly ground black pepper
- ¼ tsp. sea salt
- 2 medium ripe avocados, halved, pitted, and peeled
- 12 oz. canned albacore tuna, drained
- 8 large eggs
- ¼ c. fresh flat-leaf Italian parsley leaves, chopped

Directions:

1. Place the eggs in a saucepan and cover them with cold water.

2. Bring to a boil over medium-high heat, shut off the heat, and cover the pan with a fitted lid. Set a timer for 17 minutes. When the timer goes off, drain the hot water and pour ice water over the eggs until they are cool enough to handle. Peel the eggs and cut them into bite-size pieces.

3. In a bowl, mash the avocados. Add the eggs to the bowl, along with the tuna, lemon zest and juice, mayonnaise, parsley, salt, and black pepper; stir to combine.

4. Store the salad in an airtight container in the refrigerator for up to 4 days.

Spicy Ruby Red Salsa

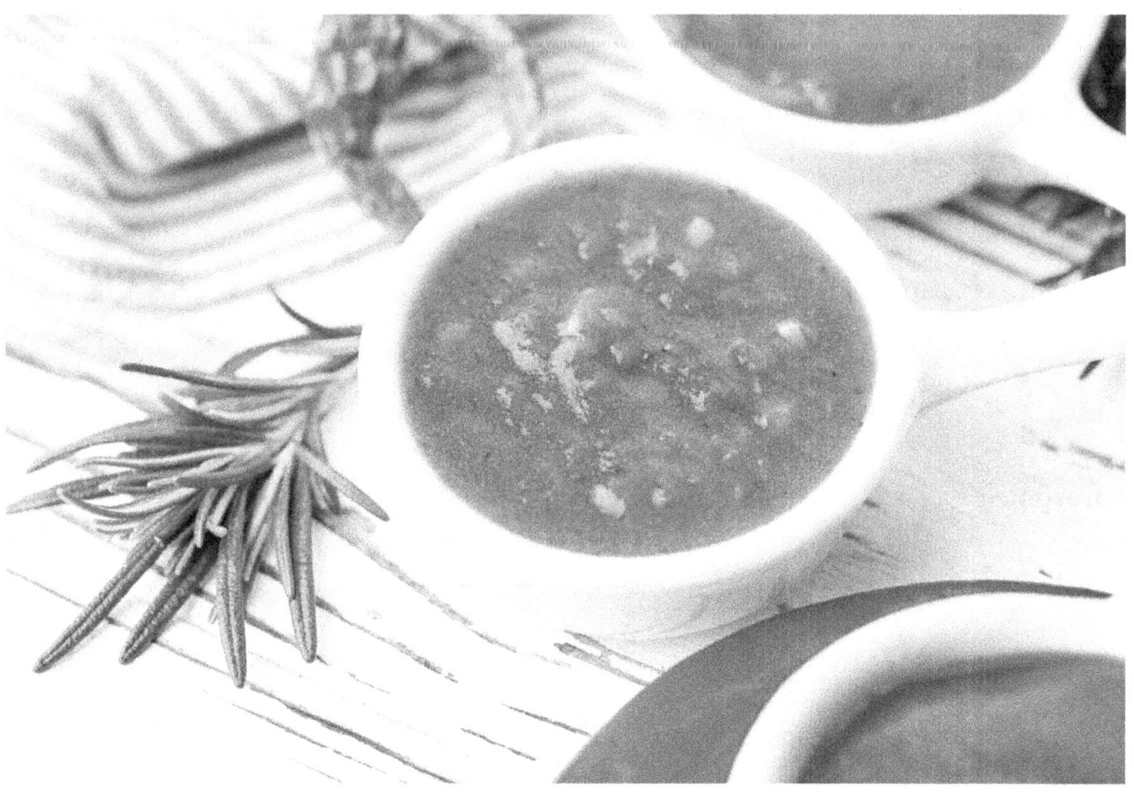

Spicy Ruby Red Salsa is a perfect combination of paprika, extra-virgin oil, tomatoes, yellow onion, and other basic ingredients. The veggie portion of this recipe is loaded with benefits that will fit everyone's nutritional needs.

Servings: 2

Cook time: 1 minute

Ingredients:

- ⅛ tsp. smoked paprika.
- ¼ tsp. kosher salt.
- 1 c. cherry tomatoes, coarsely chopped.
- 1 tbsp. extra-virgin olive oil.
- 1 tbsp. yellow onion, minced.
- 1 tsp. ground cumin.
- ⅛ tsp. cayenne pepper.
- ½ c. red peppadew peppers, quartered.
- Lime juice, ½ lime, cut into two wedges and squeezed.

Directions:

1. In a medium cup, mix all ingredients. Mix well and serve.

Chicken Stir-Fry

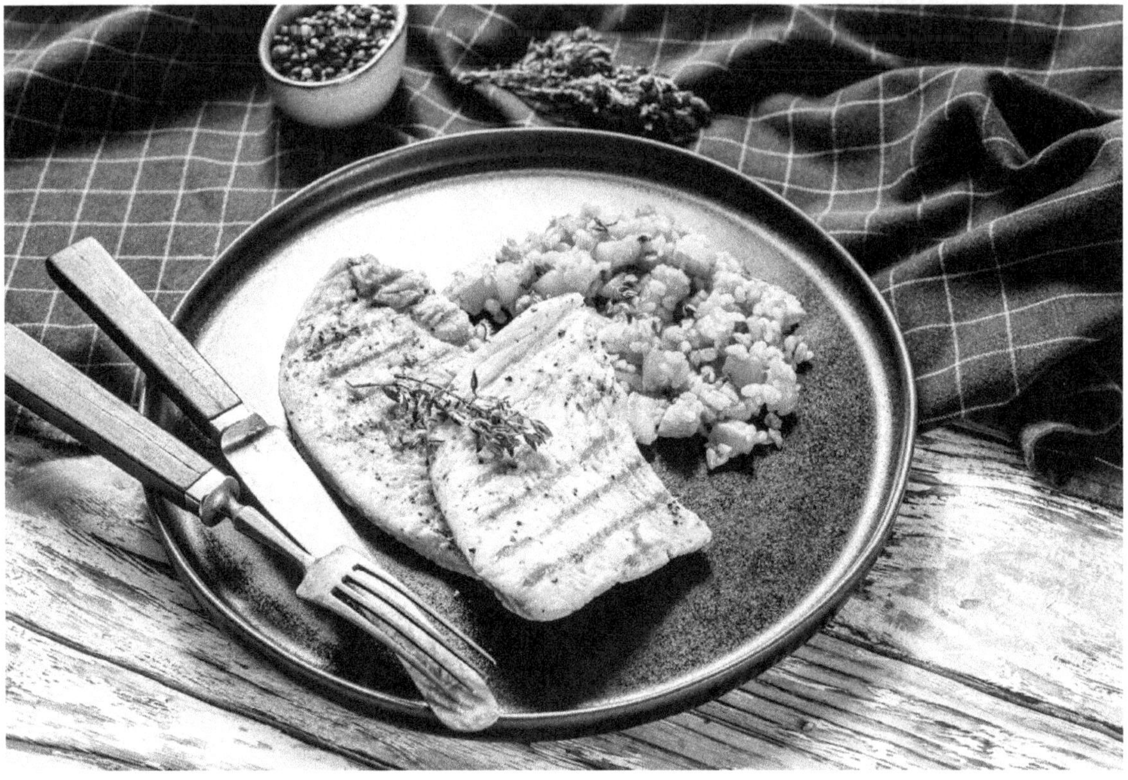

Enjoy the freshness of the incorporated veggies. With sweet sauces and other essential ingredients, you can easily prepare a sweet meal, and everyone will keep yearning for it.

Servings: 4

Cook time: 15 minutes

Ingredients

- ½ c. yellow onion, finely chopped
- ½ -lb. sirloin, thinly sliced
- 1 tbsp. balsamic vinegar
- 1 tbsp. honey
- ½-inch ginger, peeled and sliced thinly
- 2 cloves garlic, peeled and thinly sliced
- 1 bunch radishes, quartered
- ¼ tsp. salt
- 2 c. cooked quinoa
- ½ tsp. curry powder
- 1/8 tsp. Himalayan salt
- 1/8 tsp. black pepper
- ½ tsp. turmeric
- 2 tbsp. coconut oil
- 2 tbsp. tamari
- 1 c. snow peas

Directions

1. In a medium bowl, combine your spices. Add sirloin and mix well until evenly coated.

2. Heat 1 tablespoon coconut oil in a large skillet over medium-high heat. Add sirloin in an even layer, and cook undisturbed until browned on bottom, about one minute. Flip and cook for an additional thirty seconds. Remove from skillet and set aside.

3. Add 1 tablespoon of coconut oil to the skillet, reduce to low heat, and cook radishes, onion, garlic and ginger then stir frequently, until onion becomes translucent (about 6 minutes).

4. Add honey and return to medium heat; cook for about 2 minutes or until radishes are fully glazed.

5. Add balsamic vinegar and tamari then simmer until thickened (about 2 minutes).

6. Add snow peas and radish greens then season well. Continue cooking, while stirring, until greens begin to wilt.

7. Add chicken and stir until warm.

8. Serve over quinoa.

Honey Mustard Grilled Salmon

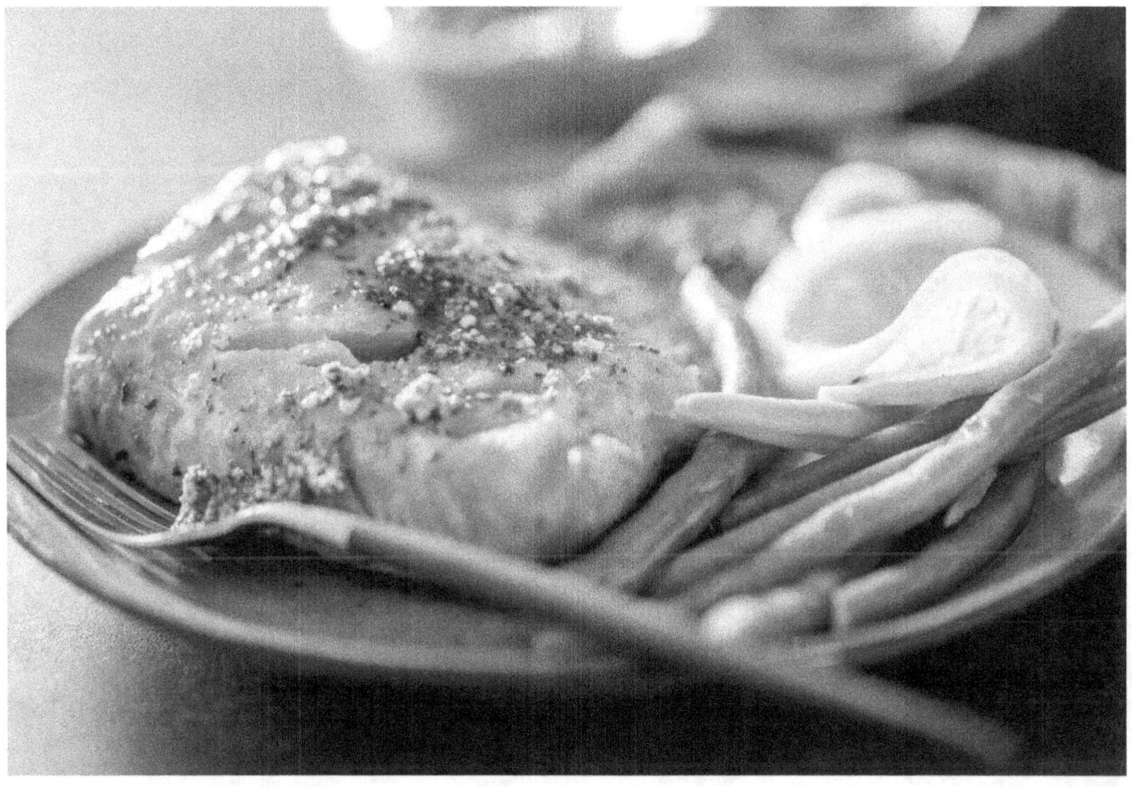

A little bit of sweetness from the honey, some hotness from the ground black pepper added onto a spicy salmon will work pretty well. Enjoy this delicacy.

Servings: 4

Cook time: 20 minutes

Ingredients:

- 1 tbsp. canola oil
- 3 tbsp. Dijon mustard
- 1 lbs. fresh salmon fillets, skin on
- ½ tsp. sea salt
- 3 tbsp. honey
- ¼ tsp. freshly ground black pepper

Directions:

1. Preheat a grill to medium heat.

2. In a small bowl, whisk together the honey and Dijon.

3. Brush the salmon with the oil and season it on both sides with salt and black pepper. Place the salmon flesh-side down on the grill and cook for 4 to 6 minutes. Flip the fillets, then brush the tops with the honey mustard mixture. Cook for another 4 to 6 minutes or until the salmon flakes easily with a fork. Serve immediately.

4. You can store the salmon in an airtight container in the refrigerator for up to 2 days. Reheat it by microwaving on high for 1 to 3 minutes until heated through.

Seafood Curry

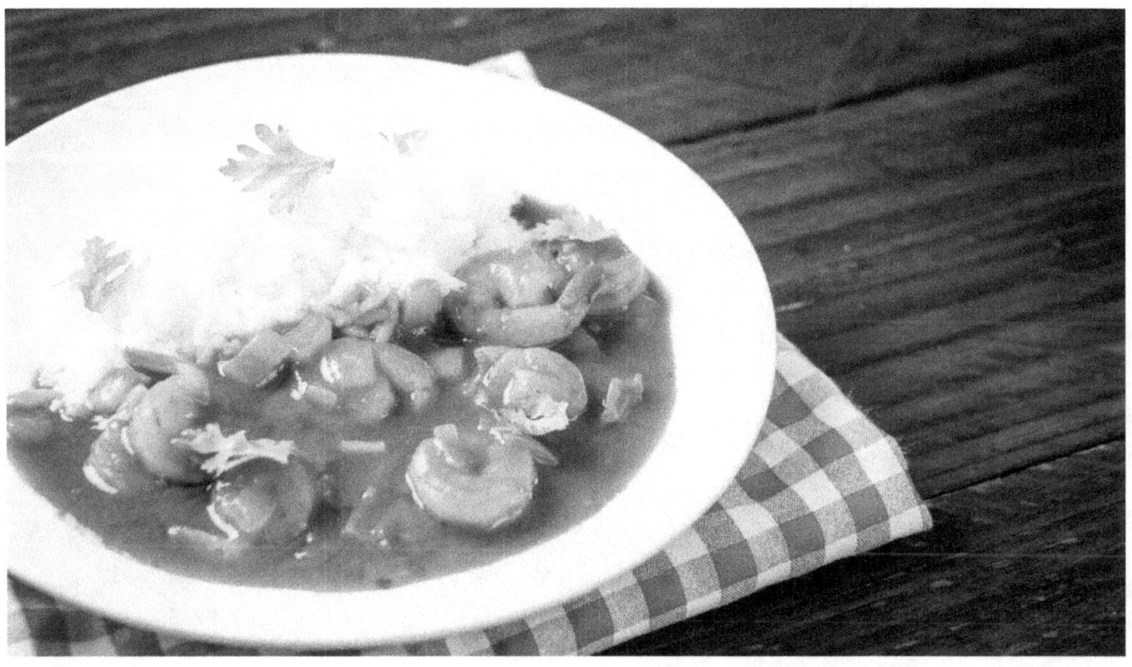

Seafood curry is packed with fresh and nutritious ingredients to ensure you enjoy the unique taste of a peeled and deveined shrimp.

Servings: 4

Cook time: 16 minutes

Ingredients

- 1 can coconut milk
- ¼ c. basil leaves
- ½ -lb. snow peas
- 2 tbsp. coconut oil
- ½ tsp. Himalayan salt
- 2 large shallots, thinly sliced
- 1 tbsp. ginger, minced
- 1 clove garlic, minced
- ¼ tsp. pepper
- 2 medium carrots
- 1 lb. shrimp, peeled and deveined
- Cooked quinoa
- ½ lime, juiced
- ½ lb. scallops
- 2 tbsp. curry powder
- 1 tsp. turmeric
- 1 c. cilantro. chopped
- 2 stems lemon grass
- 1 tbsp. maple syrup

Directions

1. In a saucepan over medium heat, sauté shallots in coconut oil until soft.

2. Add garlic, shrimp, scallops, curry powder, turmeric, and ginger, and cook for another few minutes, stirring frequently.

3. Add lemon grass and carrots, and cook for a few minutes more, turning shrimp and scallops.

4. Add maple syrup, coconut milk, salt, pepper, and lime juice, and bring to a simmer, cooking a further ten minutes. Stir in snow peas and basil.

5. Spoon curry over quinoa; garnish with cilantro.

Grilled Salmon

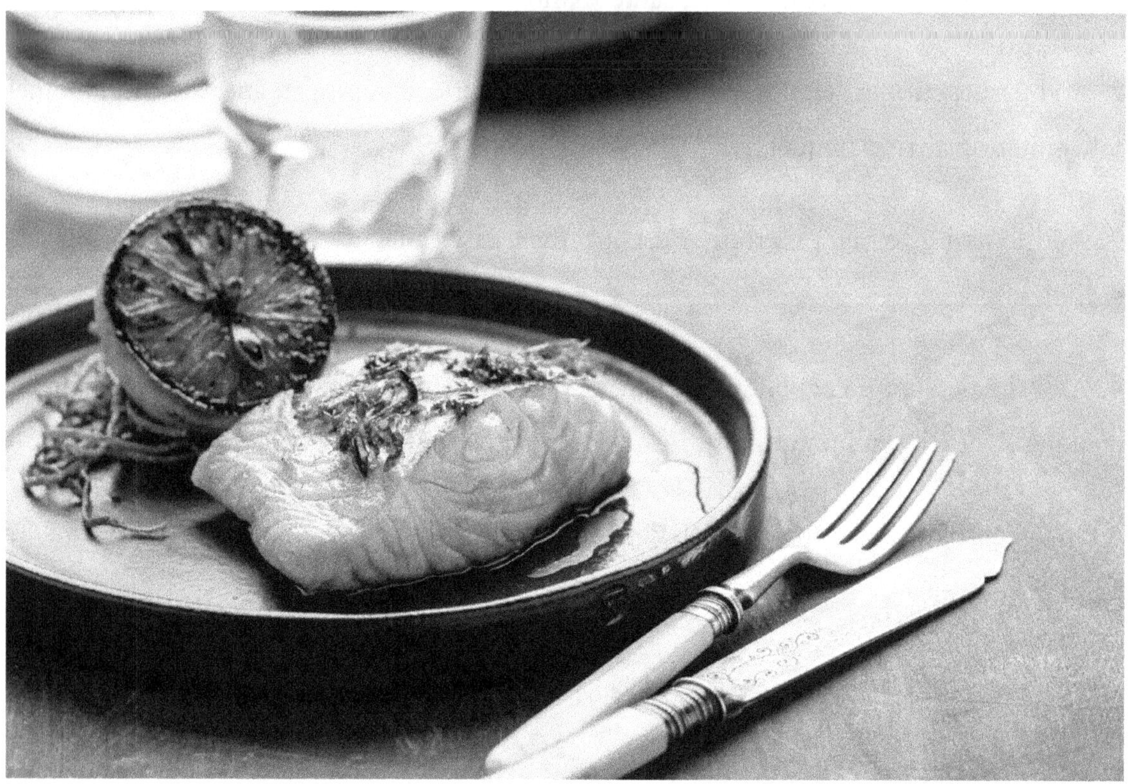

Your kids will love the unique taste of the grilled salmon. It entails white wine vinegar, some ground turmeric, wild-caught salmon, among other essential ingredients, spices, and toppings. You will enjoy it too.

Servings: 4

Cook time: 10 minutes

Ingredients:

- 1 tsp. white wine vinegar
- ½ tsp. red pepper flakes
- 8 cherry tomatoes, cut in half
- 1 garlic clove
- 2 tbsp. olive oil
- 4 wild-caught salmon filets, 6 oz. each
- ½ red onion, sliced into rings
- 1 tbsp. ground turmeric

Directions:

1. In a large bowl or a shallow baking dish, whisk together the oil, vinegar, garlic and turmeric.

2. Place the salmon in the dish and marinate the fish for at least 30 minutes in the refrigerator.

3. Flip the fillets over at least once so both sides can get coated with the oil and the spices. Heat your grill.

4. Cook the salmon on the grill for 8-10 minutes, until cooked through.

5. Top with chopped tomatoes and onions to serve.

Golden Baked Chicken

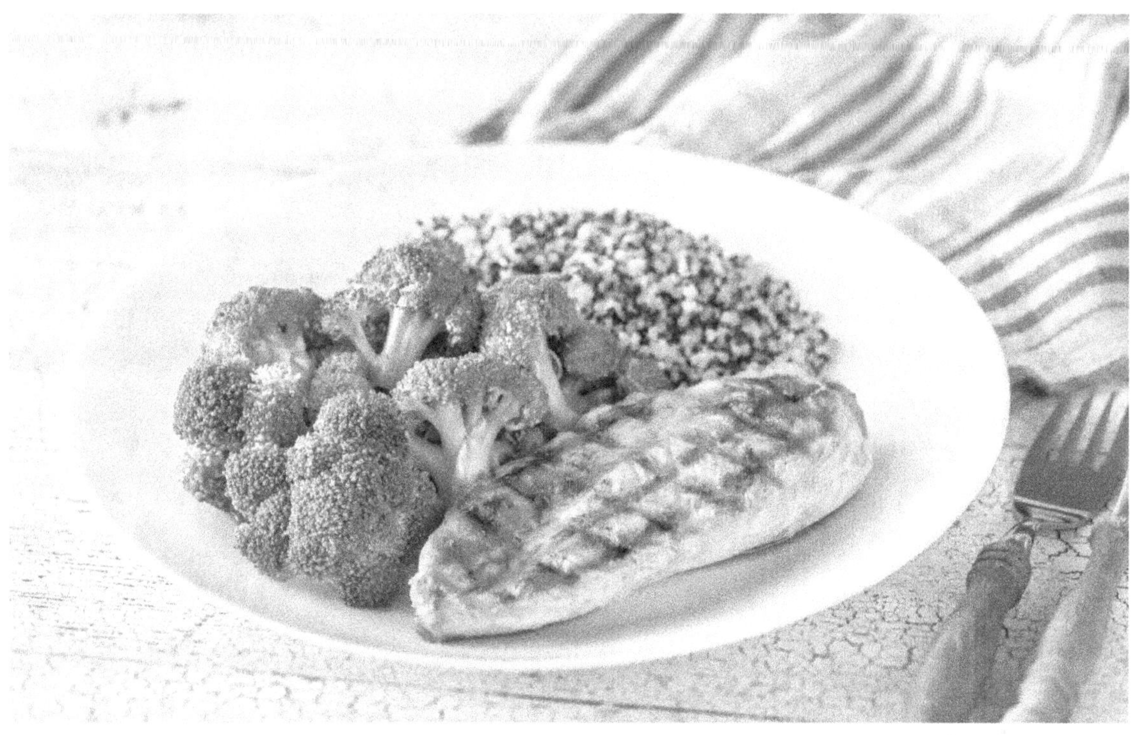

Enjoy the golden look as well as the mouth-watering taste of this wonderful delicacy. Some paprika and measured amounts of pepper give the chicken a hotter taste. Enjoy!

Servings: 4

Cook time: 45 minutes

Ingredients

- ½ tsp. turmeric
- 1 tbsp. water
- 1/3 c. blackstrap molasses
- Cooked quinoa
- 1 bunch green onions, chopped
- 2 c. mixed greens
- 1/3 c. cilantro, chopped
- 2 lbs. boneless, skinless chicken breasts
- 1/3 c. balsamic vinegar
- ¼ tsp. pepper
- 1½ tsp. red miso
- 1 tsp. rice wine
- 1-inch piece fresh ginger, grated

Directions

1. In a small pot on medium heat, add pepper, ginger, molasses and vinegar then allow to boil; lower the heat then simmer for 10 minutes.

2. Combine water, turmeric, rice wine and miso then stir into the molasses mixture. Set to cool.

3. Separate your marinade in two and set half aside. Pour the other half over your chicken and set to marinate for at least 2 hours.

4. Remove chicken from marinade and discard the used marinade. Preheat oven to 350 degrees.

5. Bake chicken, covered, in an oiled baking dish for 45 minutes or until fully cooked.

6. Serve with your quinoa and greens.

7. Top with unused marinade, cilantro and green onions.

Greek-Style Lamb Gyros

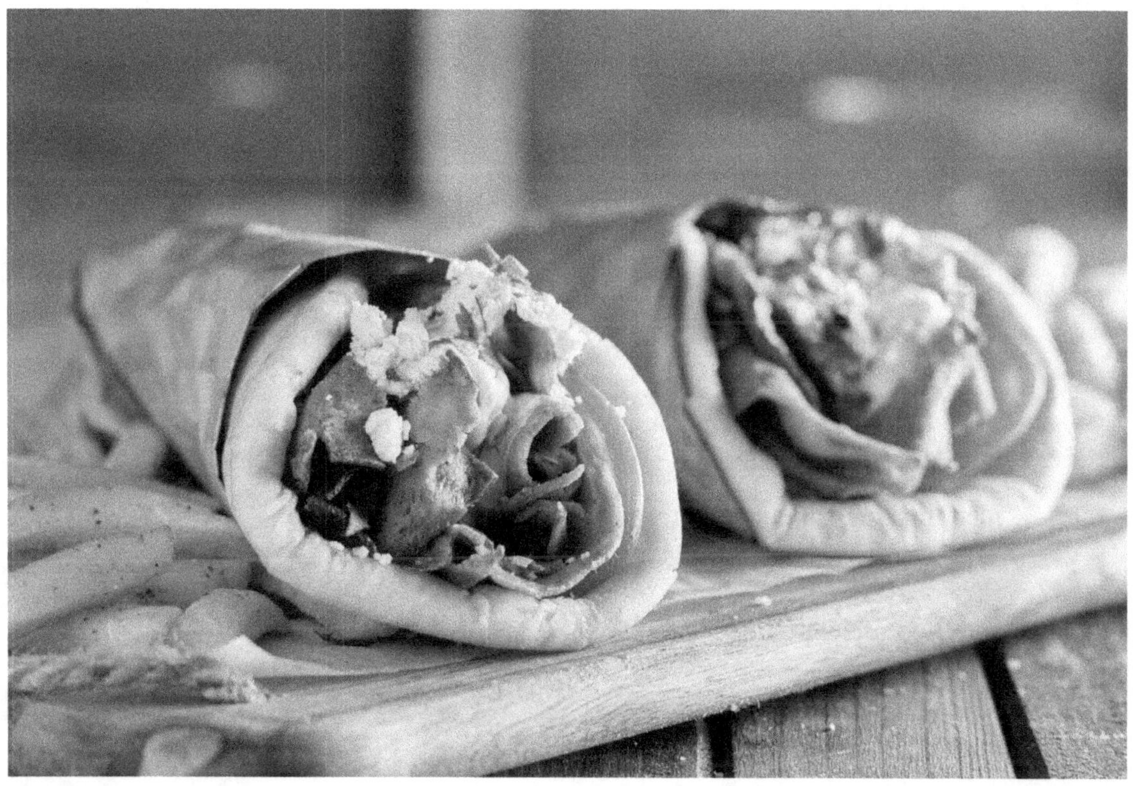

A rotisserie is mostly used for cooking a gyro. The recipe calls for some Greek style lamb with the addition of other spices and ingredients. It takes some minutes before you start enjoying the mouth-watering delicacy.

Servings: 6

Cook time: 30 minutes

Ingredients:

- 6 whole-grain pitas
- ½ medium yellow onion, diced
- ½ tsp. freshly ground black pepper
- ½ c. plain Greek yogurt
- ¼ tsp. cayenne pepper
- ¼ c. crumbled feta cheese
- 1 lb. ground lamb
- 4 garlic cloves, minced
- ½ tbsp. ground coriander
- ½ medium English cucumber, thinly sliced
- ½ tbsp. ground cumin
- 2 tsp. dried oregano
- 1 tsp. kosher salt or sea salt
- 2 tbsp. canola oil
- ¼ tsp. ground cinnamon

Directions:

1. Heat the oil in a skillet over medium heat. Add the onion and sauté for 4 to 5 minutes or until soft.

2. Add the ground lamb and sauté for 6 to 8 minutes, breaking it into small pieces with a wooden spoon, until the lamb is browned.

3. Add the garlic and sauté for 1 to 2 minutes or until fragrant. Stir in the coriander, cumin, oregano, salt, black pepper, cinnamon, cayenne (if using), and ¼ cup of water.

4. Bring the mixture to a simmer and cook just until it thickens, 3 to 5 minutes.

5. Spoon the meat mixture into the pitas, and layer with cucumber, yogurt, and feta cheese, if using.

6. Store the meat mixture in an airtight container in the refrigerator for up to 4 days. Reheat it by microwaving on high for 1 to 2 minutes or until heated through.

Mini-Meatloaf

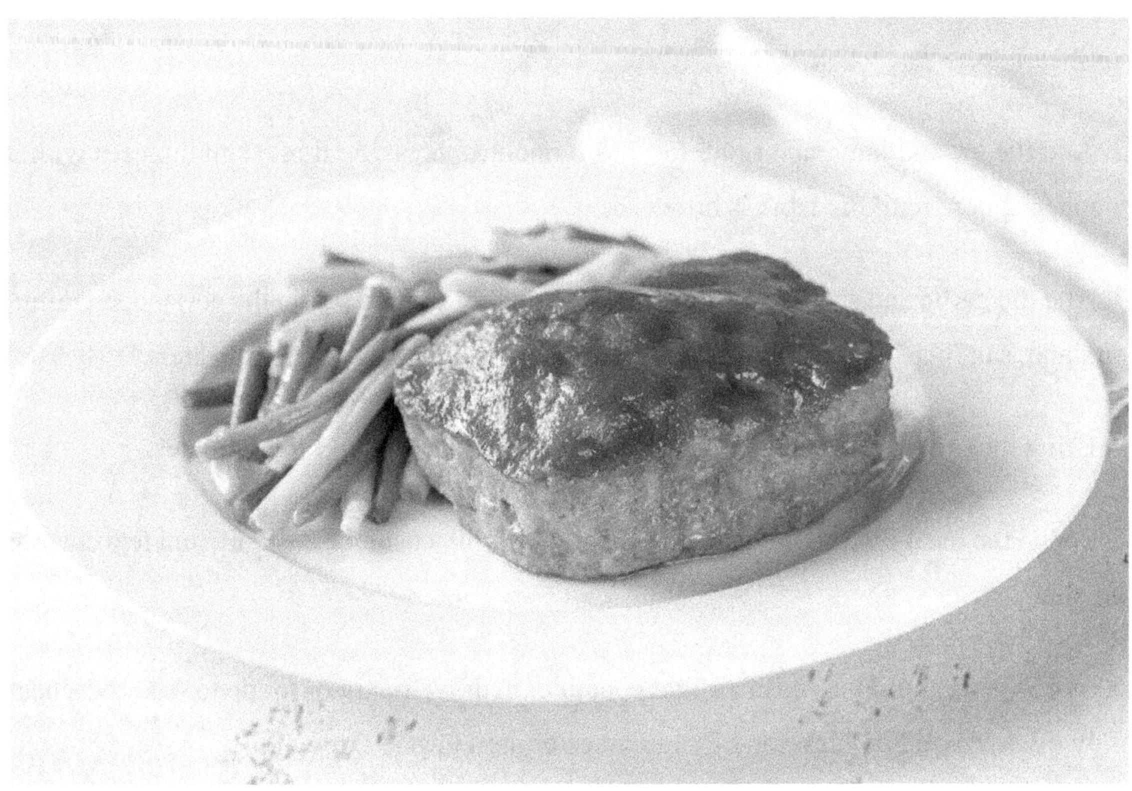

The sweetness and tenderness of the meatloaf are quite amazing. The meal entails a good number of ingredients, most of which are vital in helping you grow health-wise.

Servings: 4

Cook time: 1 hour

Ingredients

- 1½ lbs. ground turkey
- 3 cloves garlic
- ½ c. almond flour
- 2 carrots
- ¾ c. tomato sauce
- ¼ tsp. black pepper
- 1/3 c. onion
- 1 zucchini
- ½ tsp. onion powder
- 1 large egg
- 2 tbsp. coconut oil
- 2 tsp. apple cider vinegar
- 1 tsp. Himalayan salt
- 1 tsp. cumin
- 2 tbsp. fresh thyme
- ¼ tsp. Himalayan salt
- 1 tbsp. blackstrap molasses
- 1 tsp. turmeric
- 1 leaf kale
- ¼ tsp. allspice
- 1 tbsp. coconut sugar

Directions

1. Grate zucchini and carrots. Finely chop onion and kale. Press or mince garlic. Chop thyme, if using fresh.

2. Preheat oven to 350 degrees F.

3. Prepare muffin tins with liners or oil. Heat coconut oil in a large skillet; sauté onion, zucchini, and carrot until tender.

4. Add garlic and sauté a few minutes longer; allow to cool slightly.

5. Combine sautéed ingredients in a large bowl, stir in other ingredients, and mix well. Divide mixture among eight muffin tins, press.

6. Bake for forty-five minutes.

7. Combine ingredients; pour over each mini-meatloaf.

8. Bake for an additional fifteen minutes.

9. Serve mini-meatloaves with additional sauce, if desired.

Lemony Garlic Shrimp Scampi

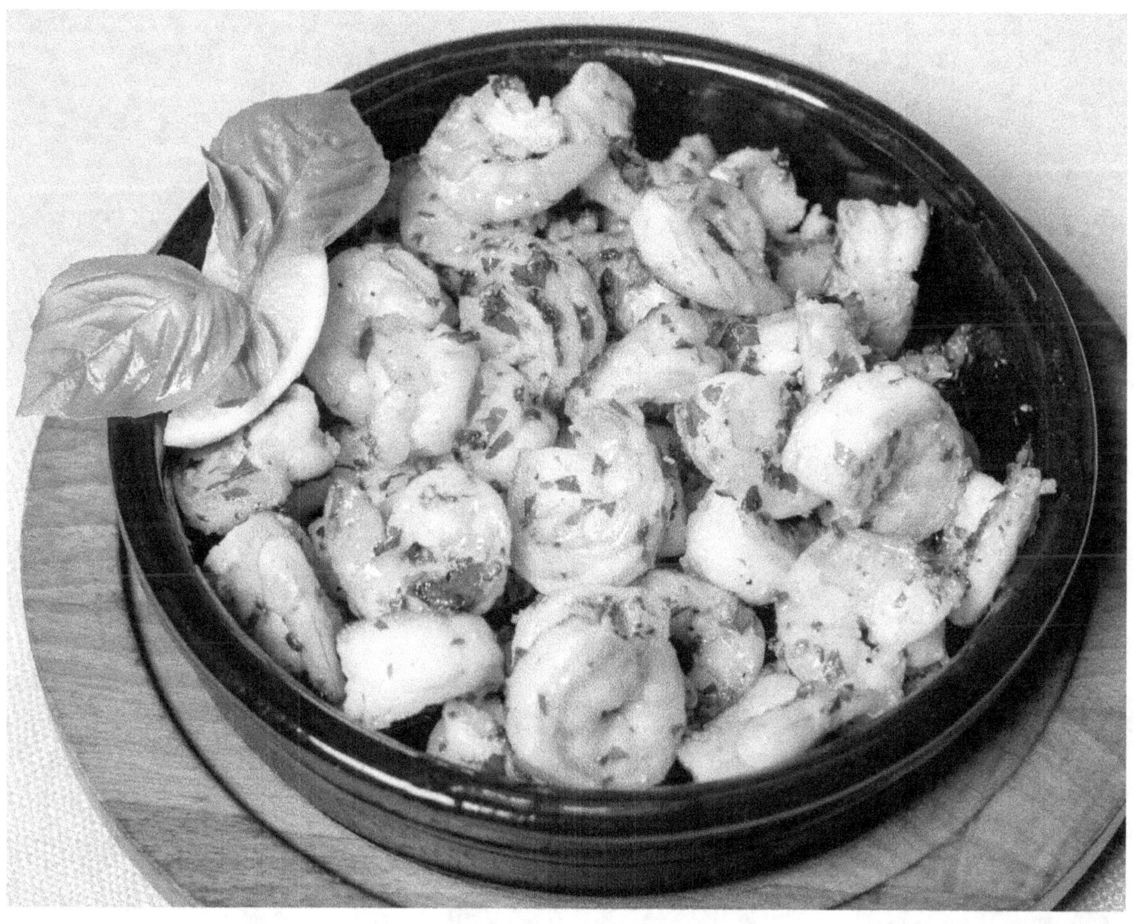

Even though shrimp scampi can be served alone, it is always a good idea to incorporate some lemony garlic taste to add to the sweetness. Vegetable ingredients play a vital role when it comes to building body health.

Servings: 6

Cook time: 20 minutes

Ingredients:

- 1 tbsp. unsalted butter
- 2 lbs. large raw shrimp, peeled and deveined, tails removed
- 1 c. dry white wine
- 3 tbsp. extra-virgin olive oil, divided
- 8 oz. whole-grain spaghetti
- ¼ c. fresh flat-leaf Italian parsley leaves, chopped
- ¼ tsp. crushed red pepper flakes
- 1 tsp. kosher salt or sea salt, divided
- 5 garlic cloves, minced
- Lemon juice and zest, ½ medium lemon

Directions:

1. Bring a large pot of water to a boil. Cook the pasta (spaghetti) according to the package directions.

2. Reserve ½ cup of the pasta water, then drain the pasta. Set the pasta aside.

3. In a large skillet, heat 1 tablespoon of the olive oil over medium heat. Add the shrimp and sprinkle with ½ teaspoon of the salt. Cook the shrimp for 2 minutes per side, until slightly crispy on the edges. Remove the shrimp and place them on a plate. Set aside.

4. Add the garlic to the skillet and sauté for 1 to 3 minutes. Add the reserved pasta water, white wine, and lemon zest and juice; and simmer until the liquid is reduced, about 2 to 3 minutes.

5. Reduce the heat and stir in the cooked shrimp, butter, remaining ½ teaspoon of salt, red pepper flakes, and chopped parsley. Cook for an additional 2 to 3 minutes or until the shrimp is fully cooked. Add the pasta and the remaining 2 tablespoons of olive oil; toss to coat. Serve immediately.

6. Store the shrimp scampi in an airtight container in the refrigerator for up to 4 days. Reheat it by microwaving on high for 1 to 3 minutes, until heated through.

Artichoke Chicken

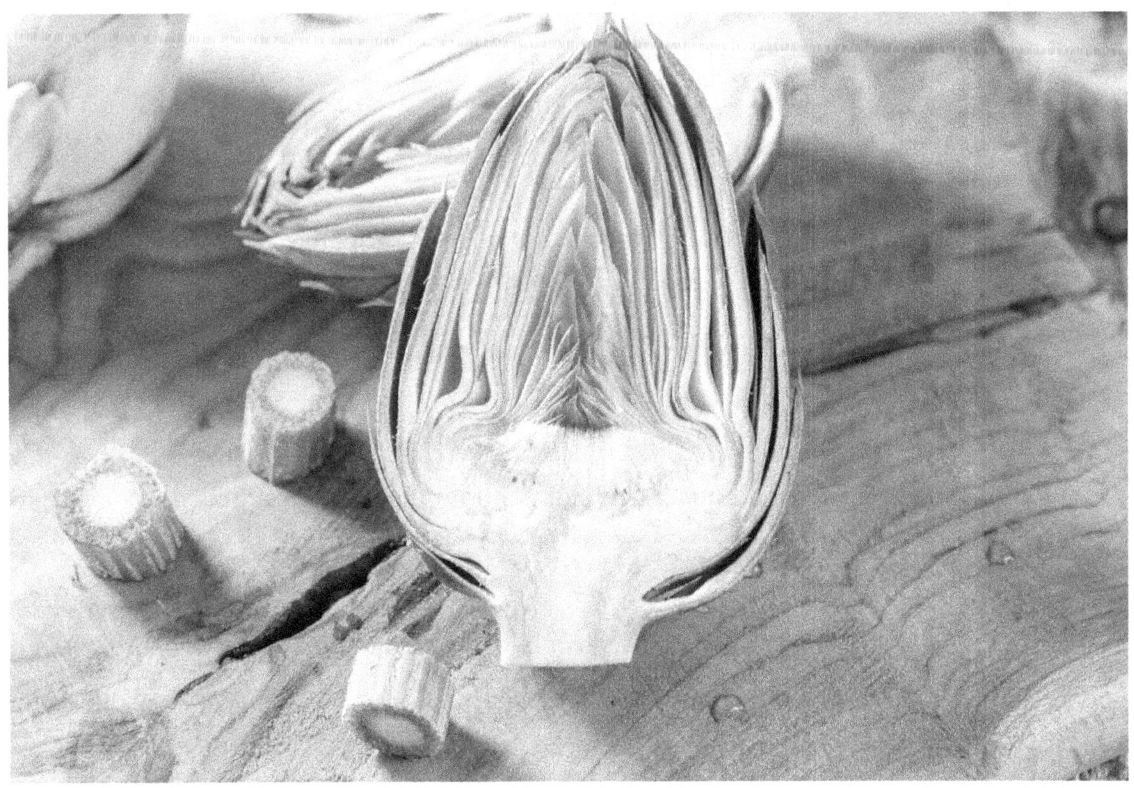

If you have been craving for some chicken that's prepared in a unique way that incorporates essential nutrients like vitamins, then you can try the artichoke chicken. It is loaded with favorite spices and ingredients that add more flavor to the taste.

Servings: 4

Cook time: 30 minutes

Ingredients:

- 2 tbsp. lemon juice
- 1 tsp. dried oregano
- ½ c. sun-dried tomatoes
- ½ tsp. freshly ground black pepper
- 2 c. water
- 1 tsp. dried rosemary
- 2 tbsp. olive oil
- 1 lb. boneless, skinless chicken breasts
- ½ c. low-sodium chicken stock
- 4 artichokes
- 2 c. baby spinach

Directions:

1. On a cutting board, using a sharp serrated knife, cut off the top third of the artichokes, as this portion is inedible. Also, cut off the bottom half of the stems.

2. Peel back the leaves until the yellow center is exposed. Using a small knife, cut away any woody bits near the base of the artichoke. Use a spoon or melon baller to remove the fibrous center of the artichoke heart.

3. In a large pot, cover the artichoke hearts with water and add the lemon juice. Cover with a lid and bring the water to a boil over medium-high heat. Cook for 20 minutes. Drain and set the artichokes aside.

4. While the artichokes are cooking, in a large and deep sauté pan or skillet, heat the olive oil on medium heat until shimmering.

5. Add the chicken breasts and cook each side for 5 to 7 minutes, or until the internal temperature reaches 165°F.

6. When the chicken is cooked through, dice the artichoke hearts and add to the pan.

7. Add the chicken stock, spinach, tomatoes, rosemary, oregano, and pepper. Cover the pan and cook for 5 minutes.

8. Serve each chicken breast on a bed of the vegetables with a drizzle of the pan sauce on top.

Mini Dill-Salmon Cakes

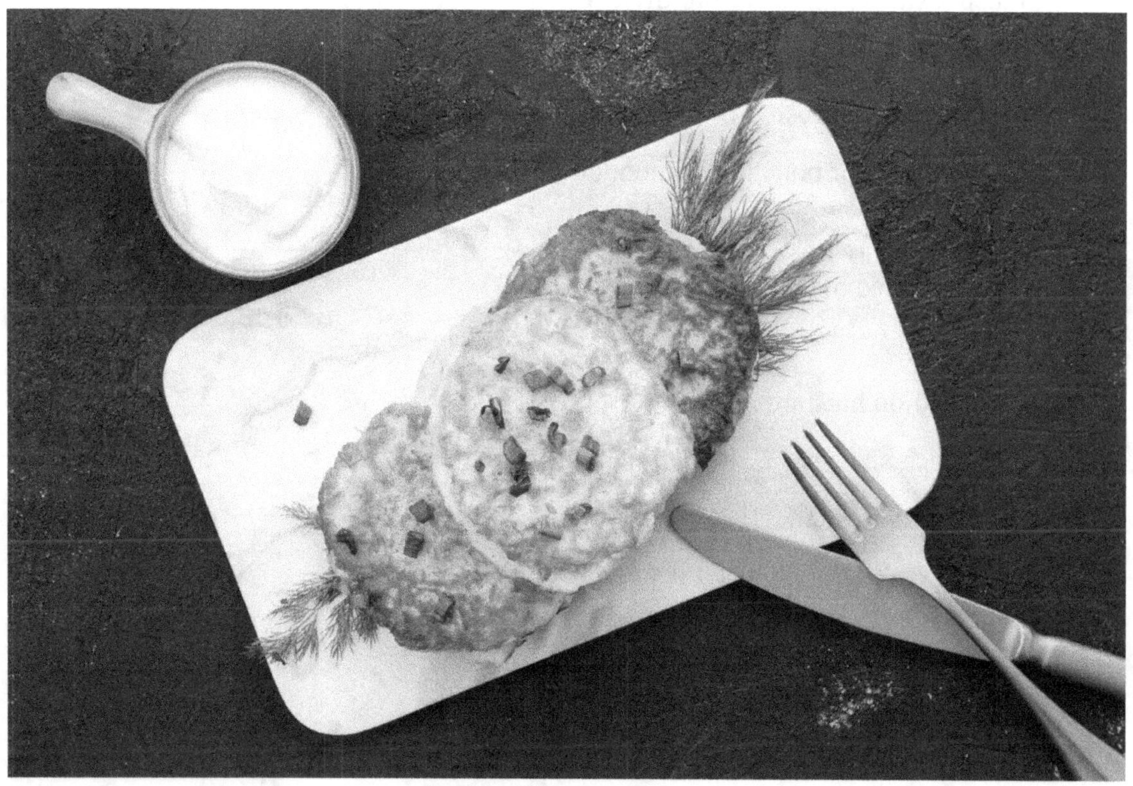

The cakes can be served as main dishes depending on their sizes. Enjoy them along with a drink of your choice.

Servings: 12

Cook time: 20 minutes

Ingredients:

- 3 tbsp. extra-virgin olive oil, divided
- ½ c. panko breadcrumbs
- 2 tbsp. chopped fresh dill
- 20 oz. canned or pouched salmon, drained
- ¾ tsp. sea salt
- ¼ tsp. crushed red pepper flakes
- 2 large eggs
- 2 tbsp. Dijon mustard
- Lime juice and zest, ½ medium lemon
- 2 tsp. dried oregano
- ½ tsp. freshly ground black pepper

Directions:

1. Place the salmon, panko, eggs, 1 tablespoon of the olive oil, Dijon mustard, dill, lemon zest and juice, oregano, salt, black pepper, and crushed red pepper flakes in a bowl; stir to combine.

2. Form the mixture into 12 (2-inch) patties.

3. Heat the remaining 2 tablespoons of olive oil in a large skillet over medium heat. Working in two batches, cook the patties for 3 to 4 minutes per side, until the exterior is browned and crispy and the patties are firm.

4. Store the salmon cakes in an airtight container in the refrigerator for up to 2 days. Reheat them by microwaving on high for 1 to 3 minutes, until heated through.

Bok Choy and Chicken Stir-Fry

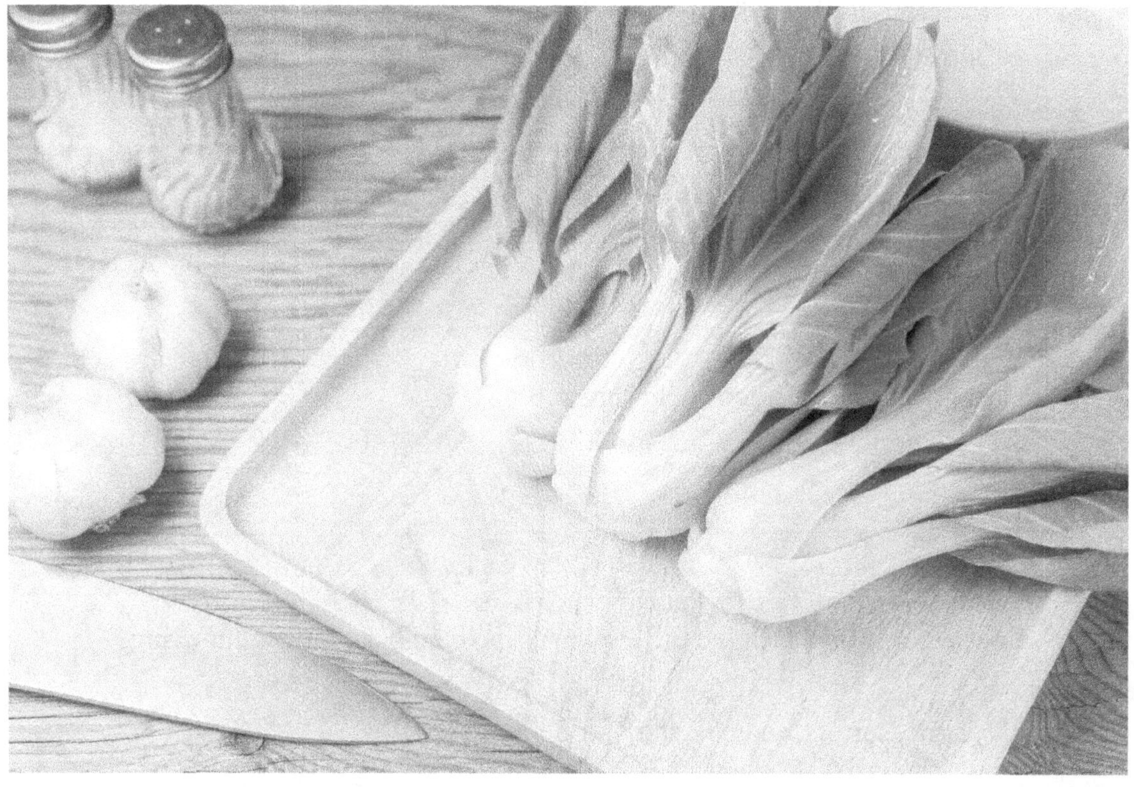

Rice or noodles can work well when served over Bok Choy and Chicken Stir-Fry. You will get anti-oxidant and anti-inflammatory benefits from this meal.

Servings: 4

Cook time: 20 minutes

Ingredients:

- 1 lb. cubed chicken breasts, boneless and skinless
- 2 tbsp. white wine vinegar
- ½ tsp. cayenne pepper
- ½ tsp. ginger, ground
- 2 tbsp. olive oil
- 1 tbsp. honey
- 2 carrots, sliced
- 1 large head bok choy, coarsely chopped
- 2 tbsp. minced garlic

Directions:

1. In a sauté pan or skillet, heat the olive oil over medium heat until shimmering.

2. Sauté the garlic, carrots, and bok choy for 5 minutes.

3. Add the chicken and cook for 5 to 7 minutes, until the chicken is cooked through.

4. While the chicken is cooking, whisk together the honey, vinegar, ginger, and cayenne pepper in a small bowl.

5. Add the sauce to the pan and stir-fry for 5 minutes. Serve.

Roasted Turkey Tenderloin and Vegetables

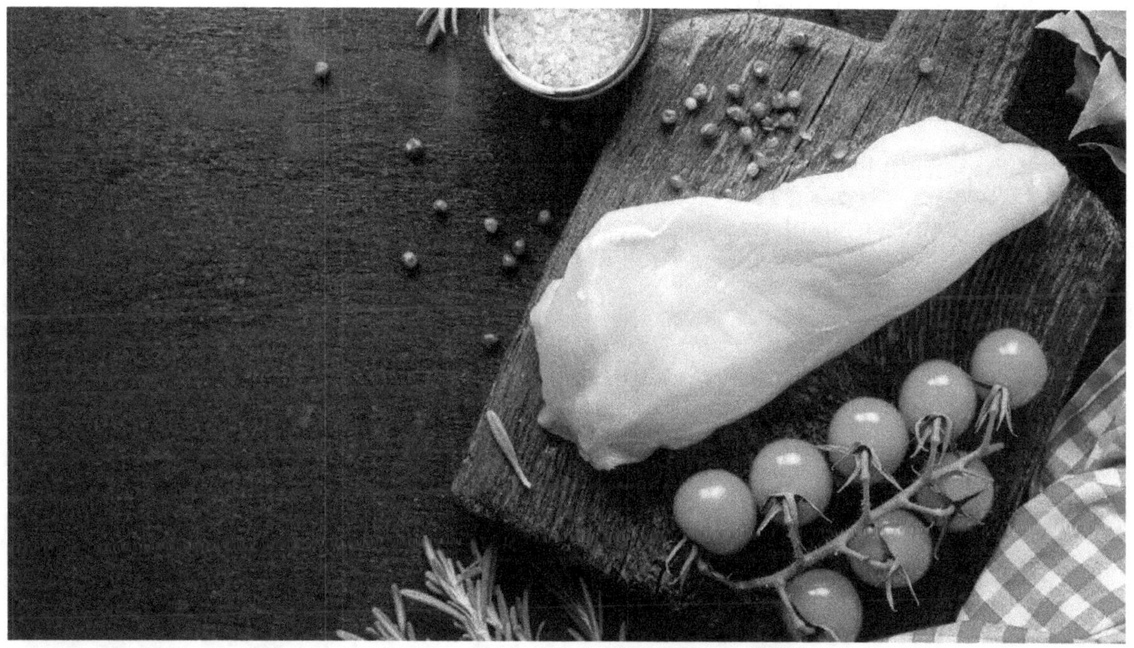

It is an easy-to-prepare meal that works as a perfect weeknight meal. Tasty seasonings, along with added toppings, make the meal sweeter. Enjoy!

Servings: 8

Cook time: 1 hour

Ingredients

- 3 lbs. turkey tenderloin
- 1 c. balsamic vinegar
- 1 tsp. turmeric
- 4 tbsp. fresh basil
- 1½ c. extra virgin olive oil
- ½ tsp. salt
- 3 tbsp. Dijon mustard
- 1 tbsp. honey
- 2 cloves garlic
- 2 sweet potatoes
- 1 head cauliflower
- 3 tbsp. extra virgin olive oil
- ¼ tsp. pepper
- ½ tsp. Himalayan salt

Directions

1. Whisk vinegar, oil, mustard, and honey. Marinate turkey in this mixture for 2 hours. Peel and mince garlic.

2. Chop cauliflower into bite-sized pieces. Thinly slice sweet potatoes.

3. Preheat oven to 350 degrees. In a medium bowl, mix oil, salt, turmeric, and garlic.

4. Place cauliflower on a rimmed cookie sheet, drizzle oil mixture over the florets, toss to coat evenly.

5. Roast, stirring occasionally, thirty-five to forty-five minutes, until golden brown and tender.

6. Put turkey and sweet potatoes in a baking dish, sprinkle with basil, salt, and pepper.

7. Cover and bake fifteen to twenty minutes or until tender.

8. Slice turkey and serve with cauliflower and sweet potatoes.

Crispy Parmesan Chicken Tenders

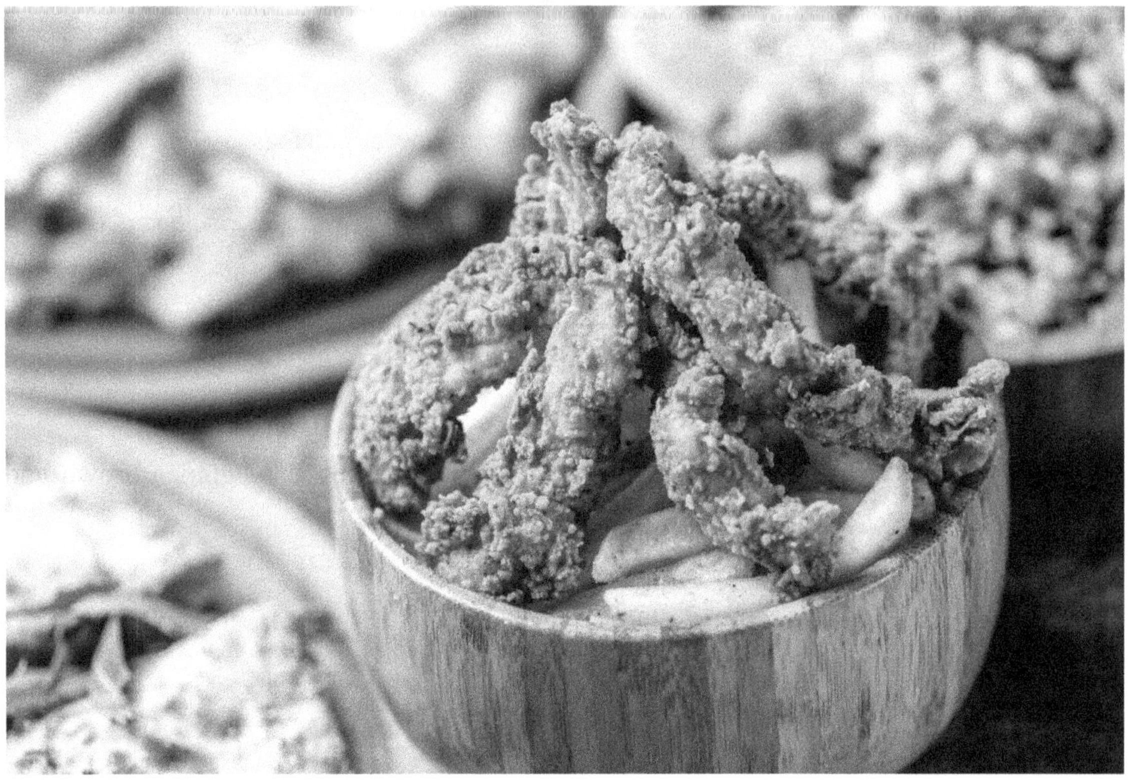

Both kids and adults love the sweetness of the crispy parmesan chicken tenders. You serve with a topping of your choice and enjoy with any other family member.

Servings: 6

Cook time: 17 minutes

Ingredients:

- 1½ c. panko breadcrumbs
- ⅓ c. freshly grated Parmesan cheese
- ½ tsp. freshly ground black pepper, divided
- Nonstick cooking spray
- 1 tsp. sea salt, divided
- ¾ c. all-purpose flour
- 2 lbs. boneless, skinless chicken breasts, cut into strips
- 4 large eggs, beaten
- 2 tbsp. Dijon mustard

Directions:

1. First, preheat the oven to 400°F. Place a wire rack inside a baking sheet and coat it with cooking spray.

2. Season the chicken breast strips with ½ teaspoon of the salt and ¼ teaspoon of the black pepper.

3. Set up 3 bowls: one with the flour, one with the beaten eggs and Dijon, and one with the panko and Parmesan. Divide the remaining ½ teaspoon salt and ¼ teaspoon black pepper among the bowls and stir each to combine.

4. Working one at a time, dip the chicken tenders into the flour, then the Egg-Dijon mixture, and then the Panko-Parmesan mixture. Place the coated chicken strips on the prepared wire rack and coat them with cooking spray.

5. Bake for 12 to 17 minutes or until the chicken is firm.

6. Store the chicken tenders in an airtight container in the refrigerator for up to 4 days. Reheat by toasting them under the broiler until crispy.

Crispy Pork and Avocado Tacos

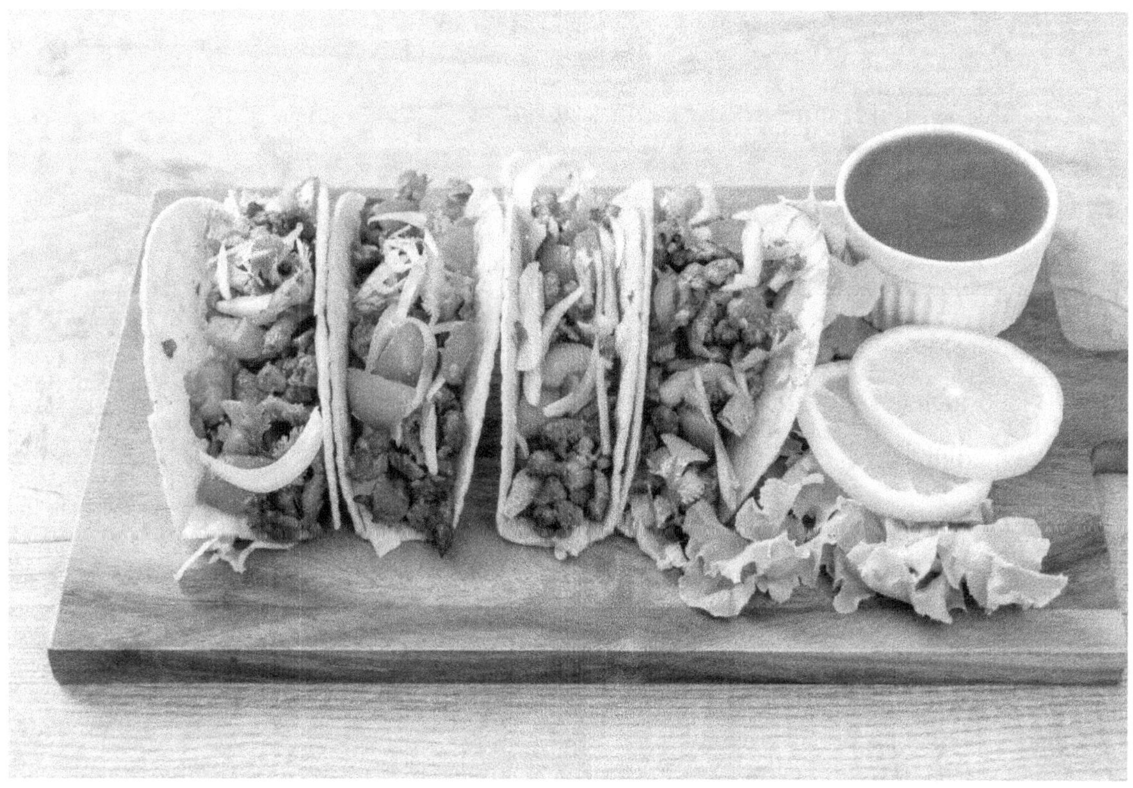

If you want to add some nutritious advantage to your main dish, then you should try some avocado along with other essential ingredients. Be sure to enjoy the spicy and delicious taste of this meal.

Servings: 8

Cook time: 3 hours

Ingredients:

- 3 tbsp. canola oil
- 2 tbsp. chili powder
- 1 tbsp. ground cumin
- 1½ tsp. sea salt
- 1½ lbs. pork shoulder, trimmed of fat
- 6 garlic cloves, sliced
- Orange juice and zest, 2 medium oranges
- 16 6-inch corn tortillas, toasted
- 2 medium limes, cut into wedges
- 1 medium onion, thinly sliced
- ¾ tsp. freshly ground black pepper
- 2 medium ripe avocados, pitted, peeled, and sliced
- ½ c. thinly sliced red cabbage

Directions:

1. Heat the oil in a Dutch oven over medium-high heat. Rub the pork shoulder with chili powder, cumin, salt, and black pepper. Sear the pork shoulder for 2 to 3 minutes per side or until a thick, browned crust forms.

2. Add the onion, garlic, and orange zest and juice to the Dutch oven. Place a lid on top and reduce the heat to medium low. Simmer for 2 to 3 hours or until the pork shoulder shreds easily with a fork. If the liquid cooks off before the pork is cooked, add 1 to 2 cups of water or stock.

3. Serve the pork in toasted corn tortillas with avocado slices, cabbage, and a squeeze of lime juice.

4. Store the pork in an airtight container in the refrigerator for up to 4 days. Reheat it by microwaving on high for 1 to 3 minutes or until heated through. Assemble the tacos just before eating.

Desserts/Snacks

The desserts here are sweet and have varied flavors that everyone will love. Furthermore, they stick to a proper nutritional guideline to ensure that every nutrient caters to the health needs of the brain as well as the body as a whole. Enjoy!

Raspberry and Banana Yogurt Ice Cream

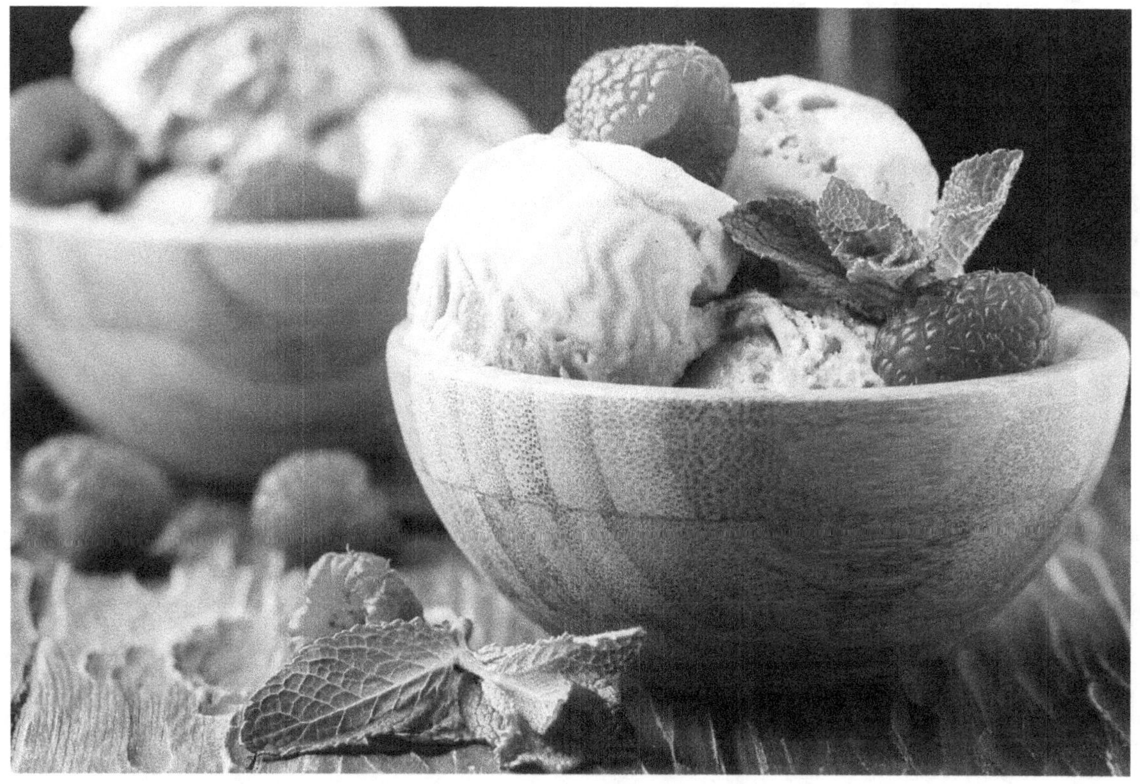

Give your kids a healthier treat by trying this ice cream. Only a few ingredients are enough to give your packed flavors. Enjoy!

Servings: 8

Cook time: 5 minutes

Ingredients:

- 1 tsp. vanilla extract
- 7 oz. raspberries, frozen
- 1 c. Greek yogurt, low-fat
- 3 bananas (large), ripe

Directions:

1. Slice the bananas into ¾" (2cm) portions and put in a Ziploc bag. Remove the excess air, and seal tightly.

2. Freeze the bananas until firm or for about 6 hours.

3. Meanwhile, use muslin or cheesecloth to line a sieve. Stand over one bowl, with the sieve well bottom clear of the bowl's base.

4. Spoon the yogurt into the cloth. Gather the cloth's ends and twist to close.

5. Put a sauce on top of the cloth and weigh it down with 2 cans (14 oz or 400g).

6. Refrigerate to drain for around 4 hours.

7. In a food processor, combine the frozen banana, raspberries, yogurt, and vanilla. Blend until evenly combined and smooth in consistency.

8. Stop occasionally and use a rubber spatula to scrape the sides.

9. Place the mixture in a container and freeze until firm or for about 6 hours.

10. Before serving, remove from the freezer for about 10 minutes.

11. If you wish to serve the yogurt individually, freeze the mixture in Popsicle molds.

Sweet Nut Mix

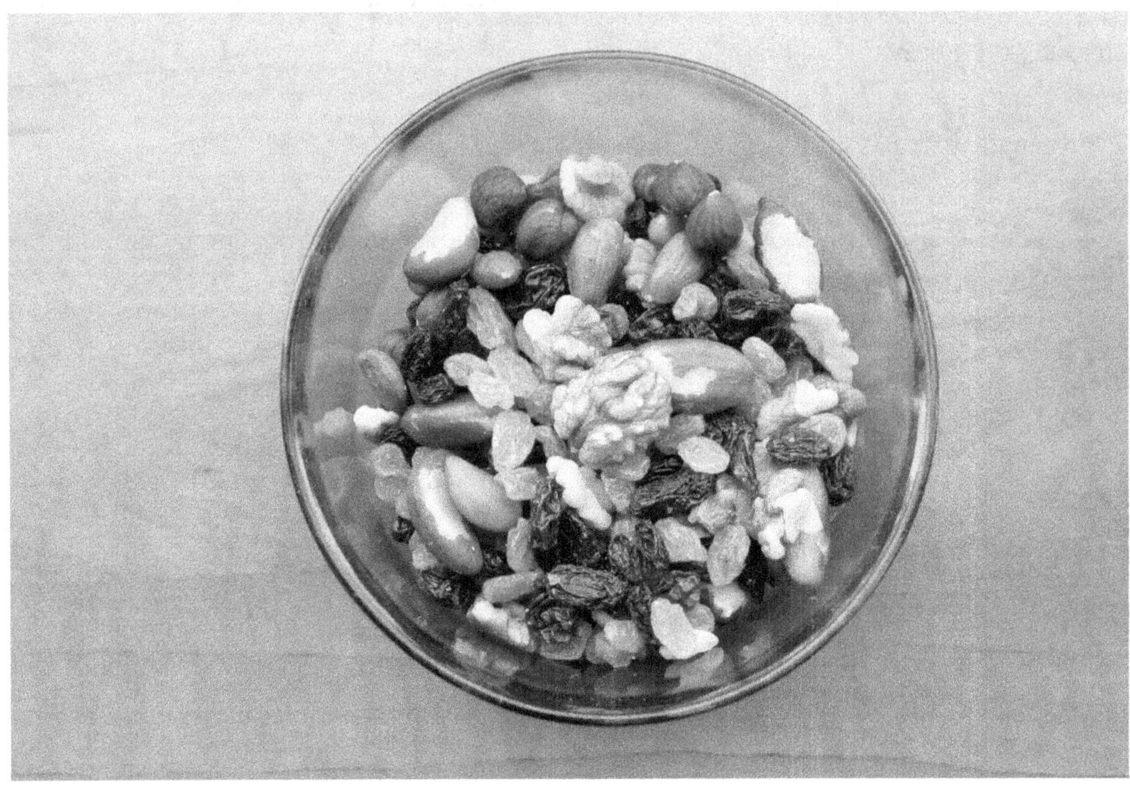

The mix of nuts is quite amazing. You will enjoy the flavors from walnuts, peanuts, pecans, hazelnuts, cranberries, and dark chocolate chips.

Servings: 4

Cook time: 10 minutes

Ingredients:

- ¼ c. unsalted hazelnuts
- ½ c. dried cranberries
- ¼ c. unsalted pecans
- ¼ c. unsalted peanuts
- ¼ c. unsalted walnuts
- ¼ c. vegan dark chocolate chips

Directions:

1. Preheat the oven to 350°F.

2. On a parchment paper–lined baking sheet, spread the nuts in one layer.

3. Roast the nuts for 8 minutes.

4. Let the nuts cool for 10 minutes.

5. Toss the nuts with the dark chocolate and dried cranberries and serve.

Dark Chocolate Bites

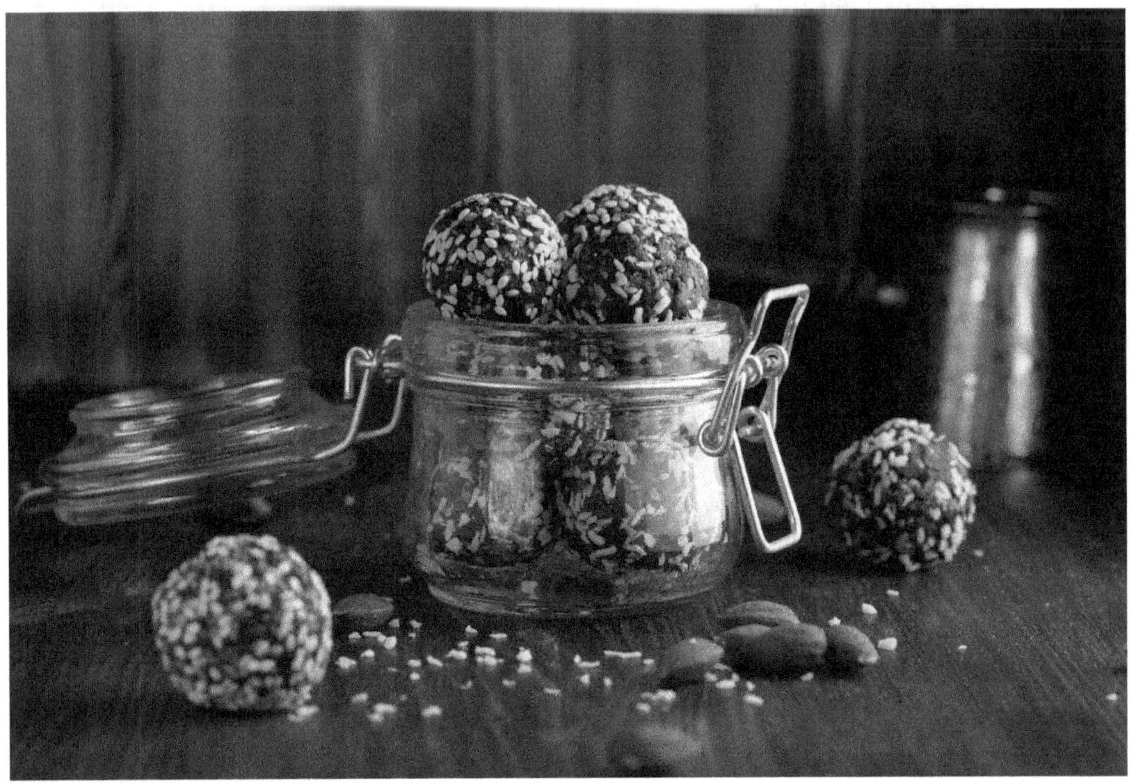

Give your kids some unforgettable moments by preparing these bites. All you need is peanut butter, cocoa powder, dark chocolate chips, vanilla extract, and old-fashioned rolled oats.

Servings: 16

Cook time: 30 minutes

Ingredients:

- 1 tsp. vanilla extract
- ¼ c. vegan dark chocolate chips, 60%-85% cacao
- ¾ c. old-fashioned rolled oats
- ¼ c. unsweetened cocoa powder
- ¾ c. peanut butter

Directions:

1. In a blender, purée the oats, nut butter, cocoa powder, and vanilla until a thick paste is made, about 30 seconds.

2. In a large bowl, combine the purée with the chocolate chips.

3. Make each bite using 2 tablespoons of the mixture. Roll into a ball and set on a plate.

4. Freeze the bites for 30 minutes.

5. Store in an airtight container in the refrigerator.

6. Serve whenever you need a sweet treat.

Creamy Avocado Cups

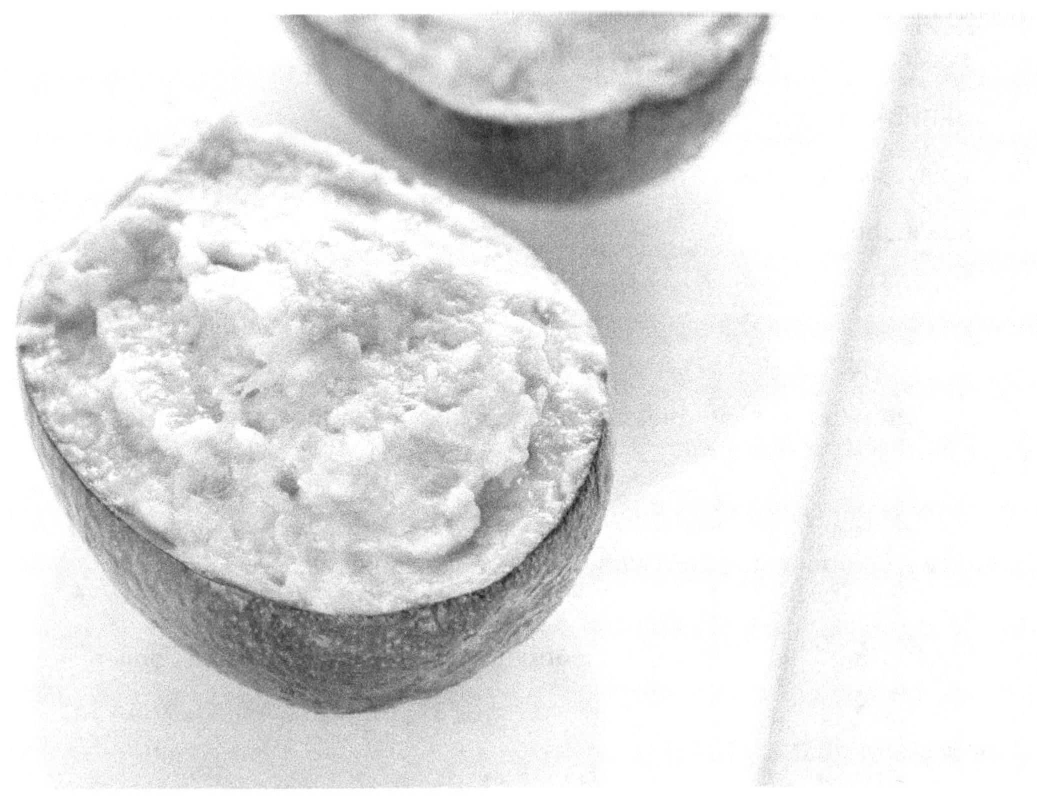

Enjoy the tasty, creamy, sweet, and delicious avocado cups. Avocado and other ingredients are packed with all the main nutrients you need for mental growth.

Servings: 4

Cook time: 37 minutes

Ingredients

- ¼ tsp. ground cumin
- 1 tbsp. reduced-fat sour cream
- 1 tbsp. chopped fresh cilantro
- 1 avocado
- 12 endive leaves
- 1 tbsp. lime juice

Directions

1. Mash the avocado. Set aside in a bowl. Put sour cream in a bowl.

2. Add lime juice, cilantro and ground cumin. Stir until just mixed.

3. Add mashed avocados and stir until well mixed.

4. Carefully place about a spoonful of the avocado mixture into each of the endive leaves.

5. Serve.

Blueberry Ice Cream

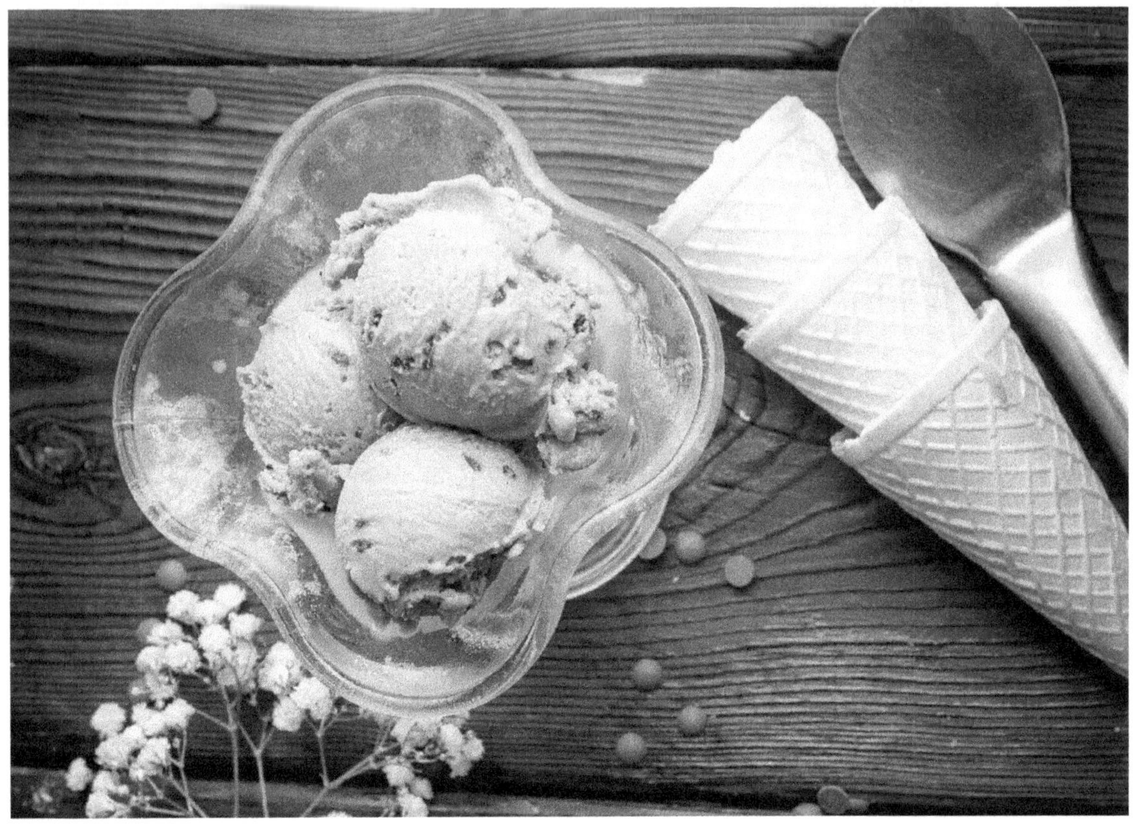

The creamy nature of this ice cream is amazing. You should try it now!

Servings: 4

Cook time: 10 minutes

Ingredients:

- 1 tsp. lemon extract
- 2 egg yolks
- 1 tsp. rosemary, minced
- 1 c. blueberries
- 14 oz. coconut milk, full-fat
- 2 tbsp. honey, raw

Directions:

1. In a food processor or blender, combine the blueberries, coconut milk, rosemary, honey, and lemon extract. Blend until you achieve a smooth consistency.

2. In a saucepan on medium-high heat, pour the mixture and add egg yolks.

3. Whisk continually until you bring the mixture to a low boil. As it starts to boil, remove the mixture and cool.

4. Transfer the blueberry mix into a bowl and cover with cling wrap. Place in the refrigerator for a minimum of 2 hours. You can also refrigerate overnight.

5. Transfer the mix into an ice cream maker and churn until you reach the right consistency. Scoop out the ice cream immediately.

6. You may store in the freezer or serve the ice cream immediately.

Chia Sesame Balls

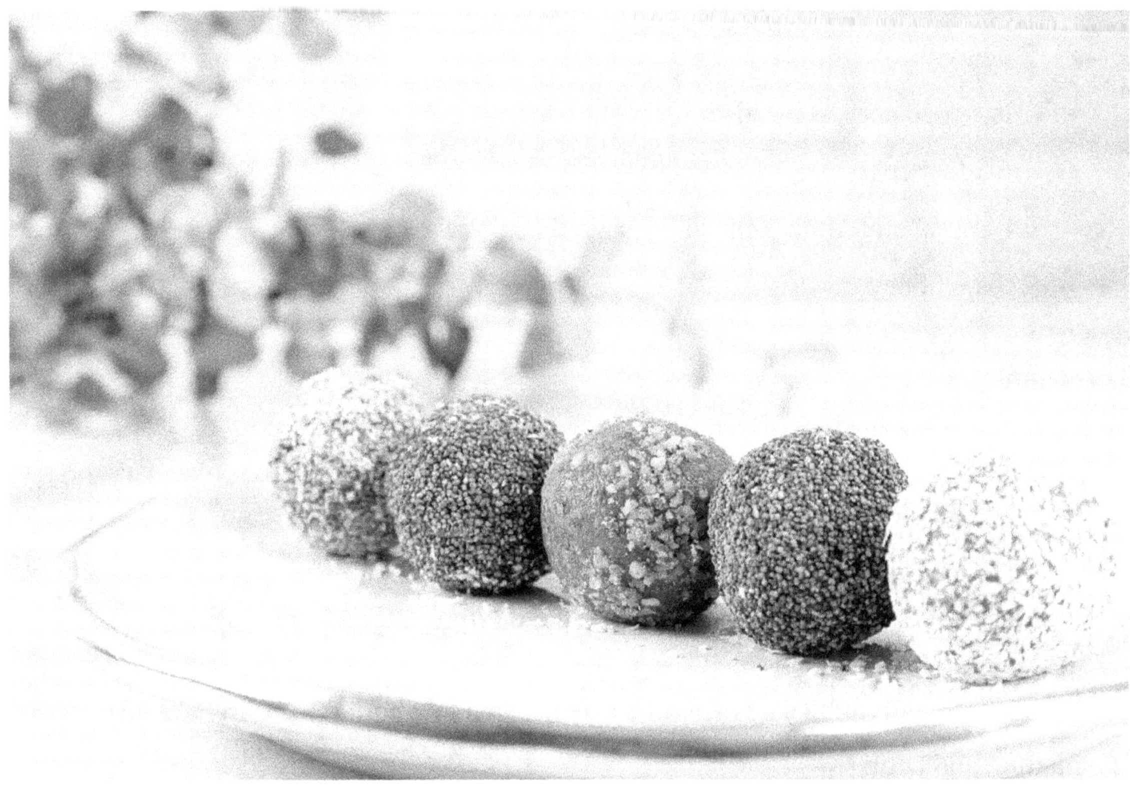

Many people love sesame balls because they are easy to prepare and have a range of nutritional and health benefits. You will enjoy them too.

Servings: 2

Cook time: 4 minutes

Ingredients

- 1 tbsp. rice malt syrup
- 2 tbsp. sesame seeds, toasted
- 1/3 c. toasted macadamias
- 1 c. pitted dried dates
- 1/3 cup dry roasted cashews
- 2 tbsp. white chia seeds

Directions

1. Place half of the sesame seeds, macadamia, cashews, chia seeds, dates and rice malt syrup in a blender or food processor.

2. Pulse the ingredients until a well-mixed, paste-like, thick and smooth mixture is formed.

3. Transfer the mixture into a shallow dish.

4. Place the remaining sesame seeds on a plate. Scoop out 2 tablespoons of the nut-seeds mixture. Roll into balls.

5. Coat the balls by rolling on the sesame seeds.

6. Place the coated balls on a plate.

7. Chill to set the balls in the refrigerator.

8. Serve once firm.

Popcorn Nut Mix

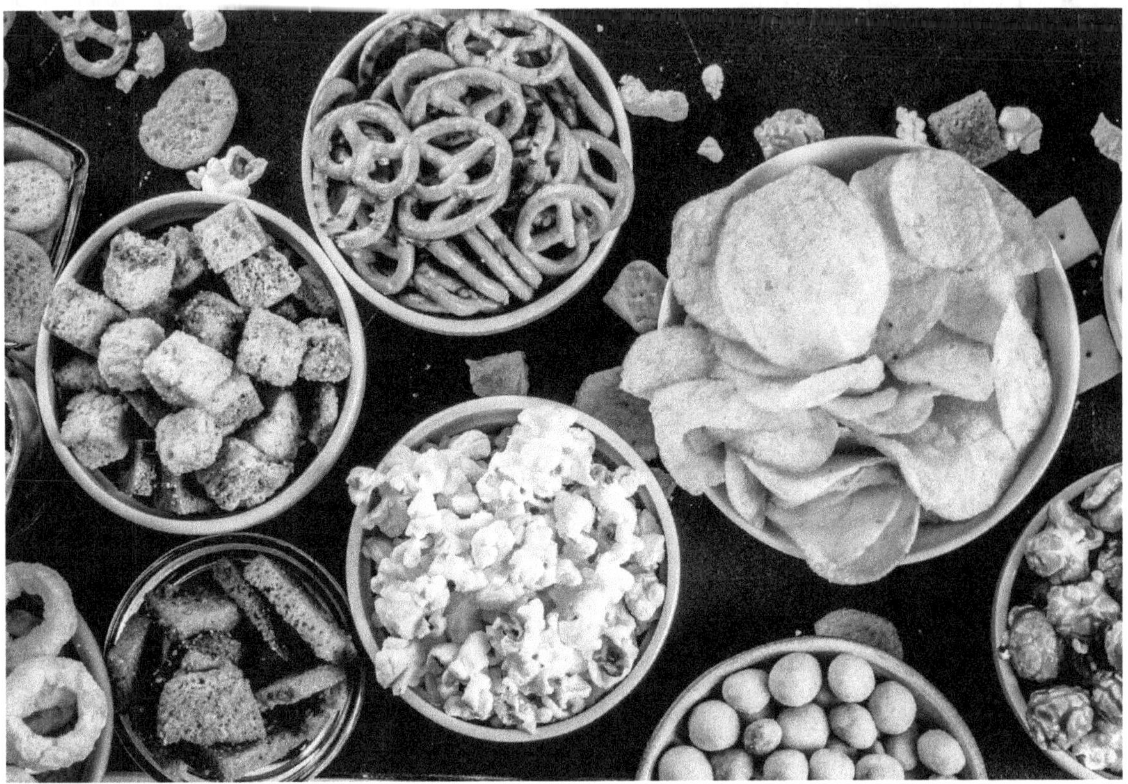

In about 5 minutes, your mix of popcorn and nuts will be ready. Enjoy the sweetness from essential ingredients such as almonds and rosemary by making this recipe.

Servings: 4

Cook time: 5 minutes

Ingredients:

- 1 tbsp. dried rosemary
- ¼ tsp. garlic powder
- 2 tbsp. olive oil
- 1 c. almonds
- ½ c. popcorn kernels
- ¼ tsp. salt

Directions:

1. In a large stockpot, heat the olive oil on medium heat until shimmering.

2. Add the popcorn kernels and cover the stockpot.

3. The kernels will pop for 4 to 5 minutes. Listen closely. When the popping slows to only every few seconds, your popcorn is done.

4. Toss the popcorn and nuts together with the seasonings and serve.

Green Juice

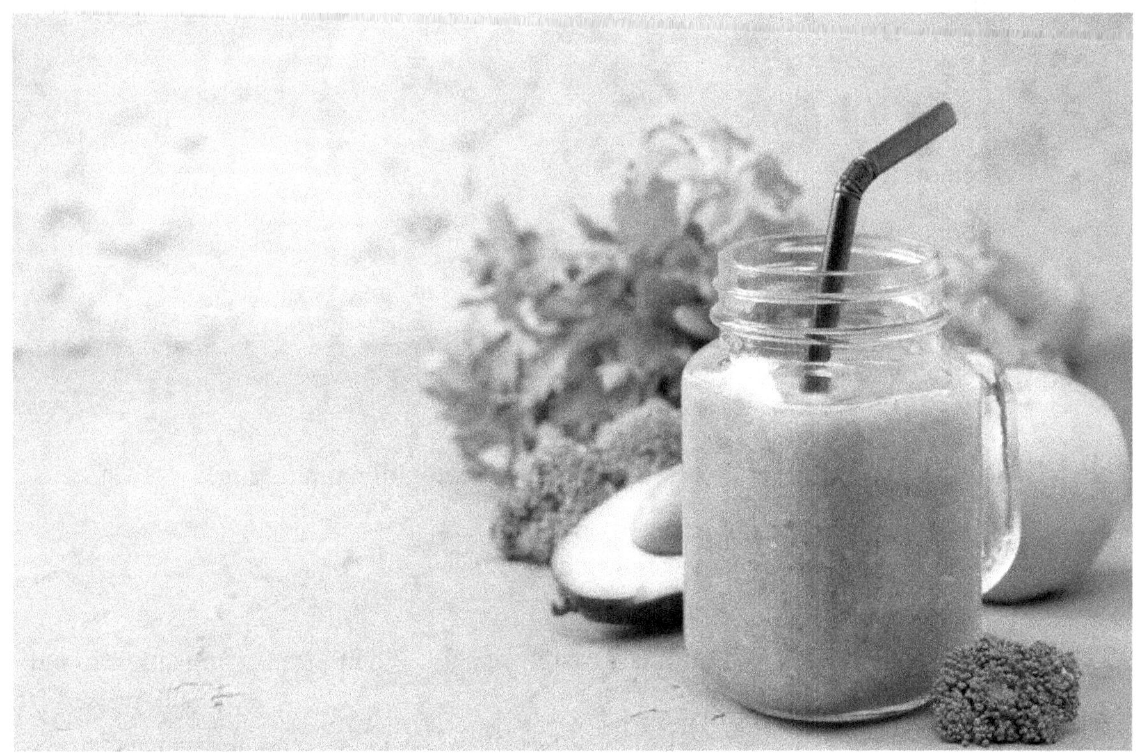

Just like any other juice, Green juice is easy to prepare and only entails a few ingredients. Enjoy a drink of your choice!

Servings: 4

Cook time: 20 minutes

Ingredients:

- 2 c. water
- 2 Granny Smith apples, cored
- 2 bunches parsley
- 2 cucumbers
- 4 celery stalks
- 2 c. spinach, packed

Directions:

1. In a blender, blend all the ingredients on high, or on the smoothie setting for 30 to 60 seconds.

2. Over a large bowl, strain the juice using cheesecloth or a fine-mesh strainer. Squeeze as much juice as you can out of the pulp by tightly wringing the cheesecloth or by repeatedly mashing the pulp into the strainer.

3. Discard the pulp and serve the reserved juice.

Kale Chips

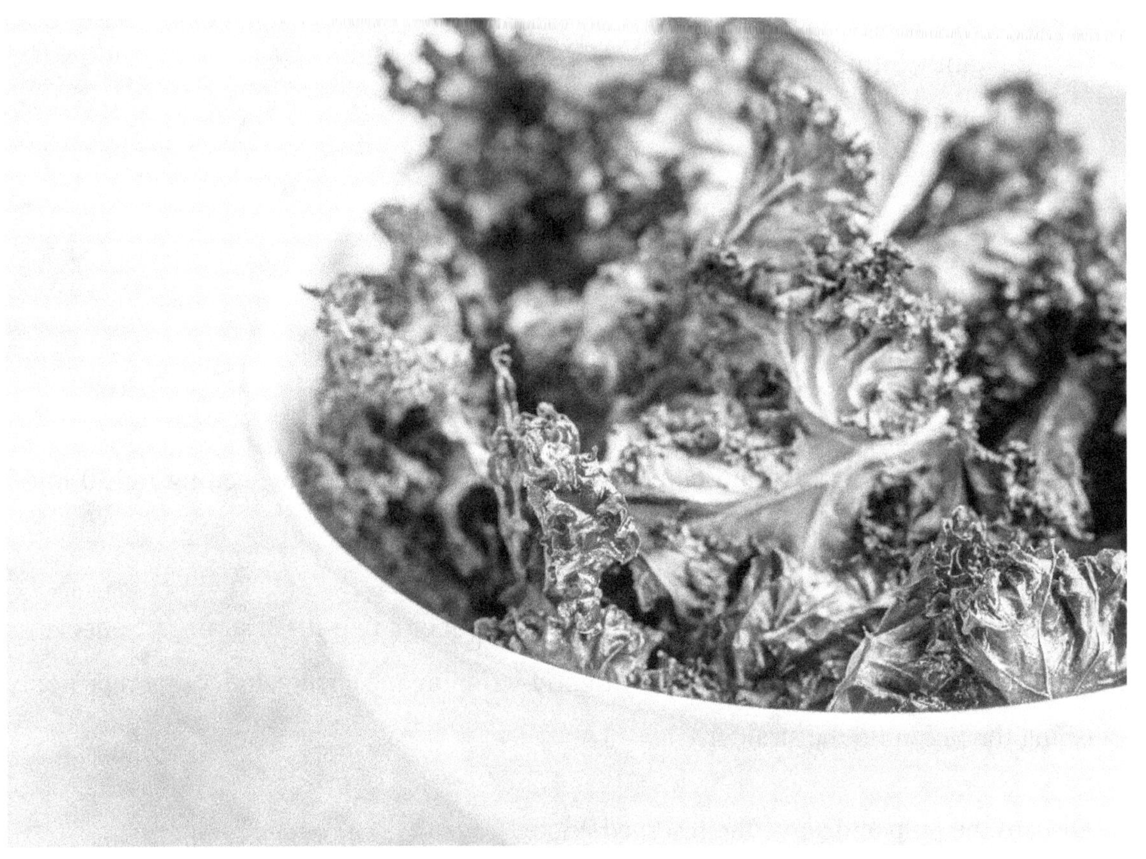

A healthier alternative for you is kale chips. Just in 20 minutes, you'll enjoy the taste of these chips.

Servings: 4

Cook time: 20 minutes

Ingredients:

- ¼ tsp. freshly ground black pepper
- 1 tbsp. olive oil
- 1 bunch fresh kale, rinsed and dried

Directions:

1. Preheat the oven to 225°F.

2. Remove the kale leaves from the woody stems and cut into large "chip" sizes.

3. Combine the kale, olive oil, and black pepper in a gallon zip-top bag.

4. Seal and shake vigorously to ensure the oil and pepper reach every nook and cranny of the kale leaves.

5. Place on a baking sheet in a single layer and bake for 10 minutes.

6. Flip the kale chips and bake for another 10 minutes. Watch the kale chips and remove before they begin to burn.

7. Serve while warm.

Coconut, Chia, Chocolate Cookies

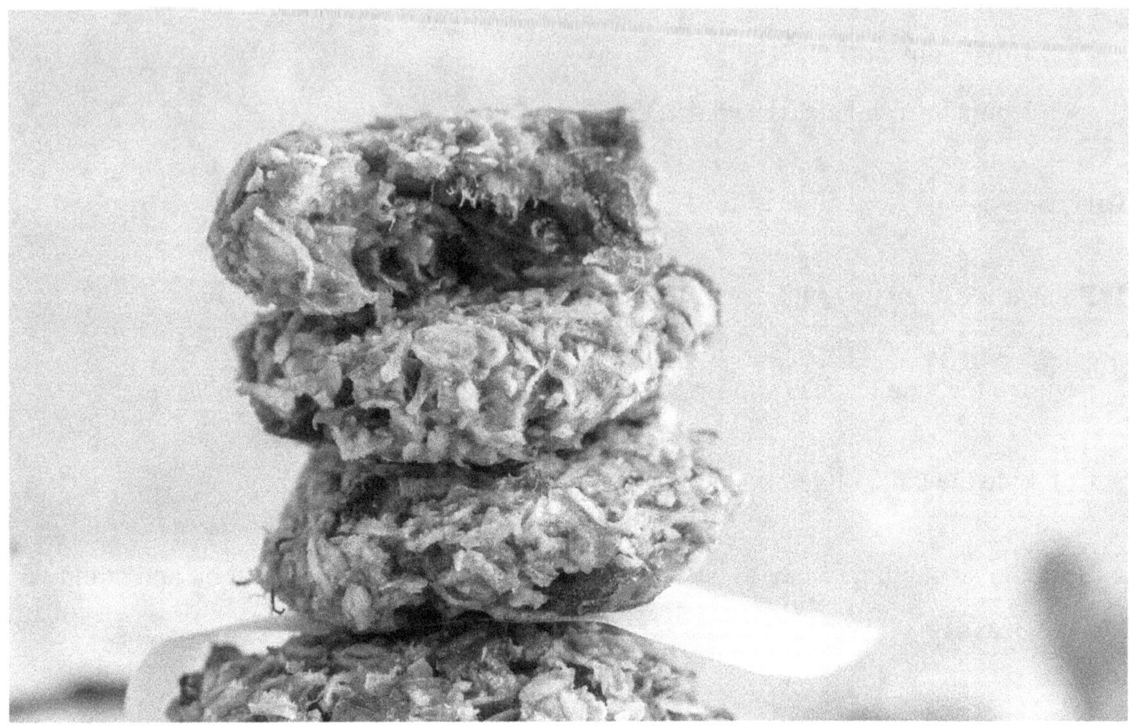

If you need energy-rich and nutrient-rich cookies, you can always opt for the coconut, chia, chocolate cookies. The recipe entails a few ingredients that are quite vital for your health.

Servings: 24

Cook time: 5 minutes

Ingredients:

- ½ c. coconut, shredded
- 1 tbsp. chia seeds
- ½ c. walnuts
- 2 tbsp. cocoa powder, raw
- 7 oz. dates, pitted
- 1 tsp. vanilla extract

Directions:

1. Preheat oven to 350° F (180°C).

2. On a baking tray, spread out the walnuts and bake until toasted lightly, or for 4 to 5 minutes. Cool the walnuts on a plate, then chop roughly.

3. In a food processor, add the dates, cocoa powder, coconut, vanilla, 1/3 of the walnuts, and chia seeds. Process until the ingredients are combined well.

4. In a bowl, put the rest of the chopping walnuts. Roll a heaped teaspoon of the chocolate mix into a ball.

5. Flatten slightly, then press gently the top into the walnuts. Do the same with the rest of the mixture.

6. Place the cookies in one layer in a container. Chill until the cookies harden.

7. You can refrigerate the cookies for about 2 weeks.

Roasted Chickpeas

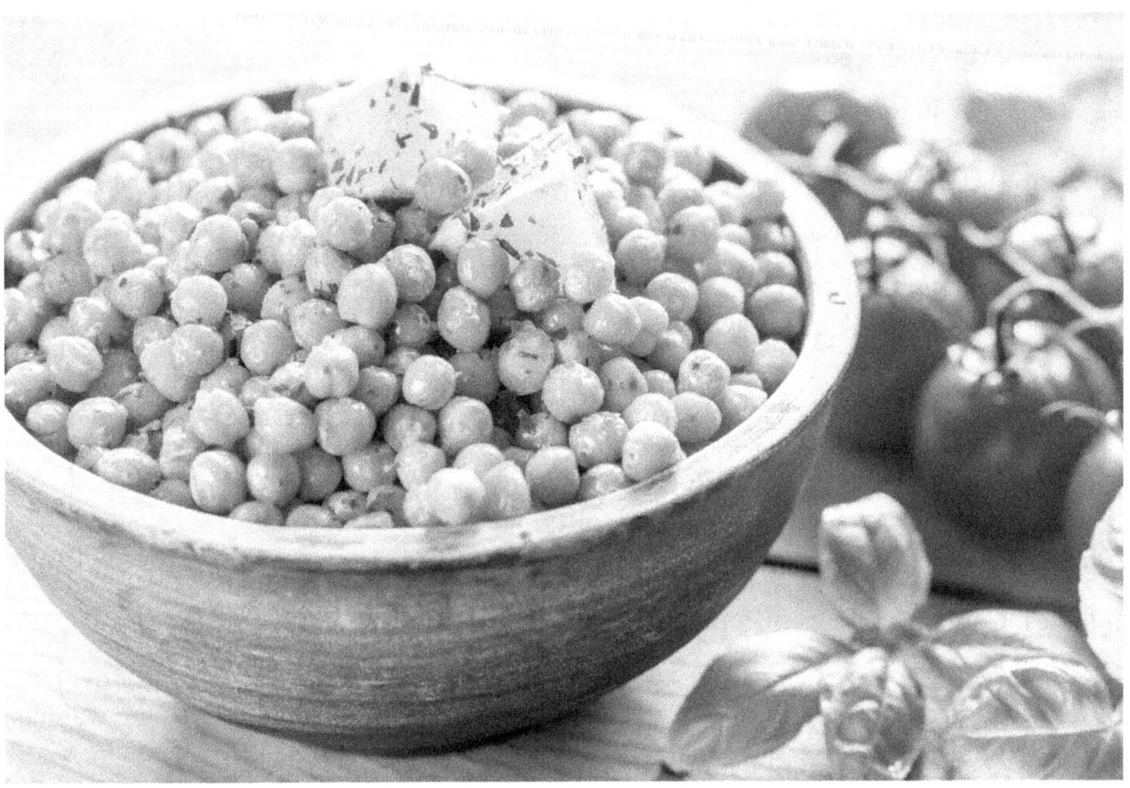

The meal is rich in nutrients such as proteins and entails a few ingredients. It is easy to prepare.

Servings: 4

Cook time: 45 minutes

Ingredients:

- ¼ tsp. garlic powder
- 15 oz. chickpeas, drained, rinsed, and blotted dry
- ¼ tsp. chili powder
- 1 tbsp. olive oil

Directions:

1. Preheat the oven to 450°F.

2. In a large bowl, toss the chickpeas in the olive oil.

3. On a parchment paper–lined baking sheet, spread the chickpeas out in one layer.

4. Roast the chickpeas for 45 minutes. Check the chickpeas at 30 minutes and monitor closely to prevent burning.

5. Let the chickpeas cool for 10 minutes.

6. Toss the chickpeas in the seasonings and serve.

Berry "nice cream"

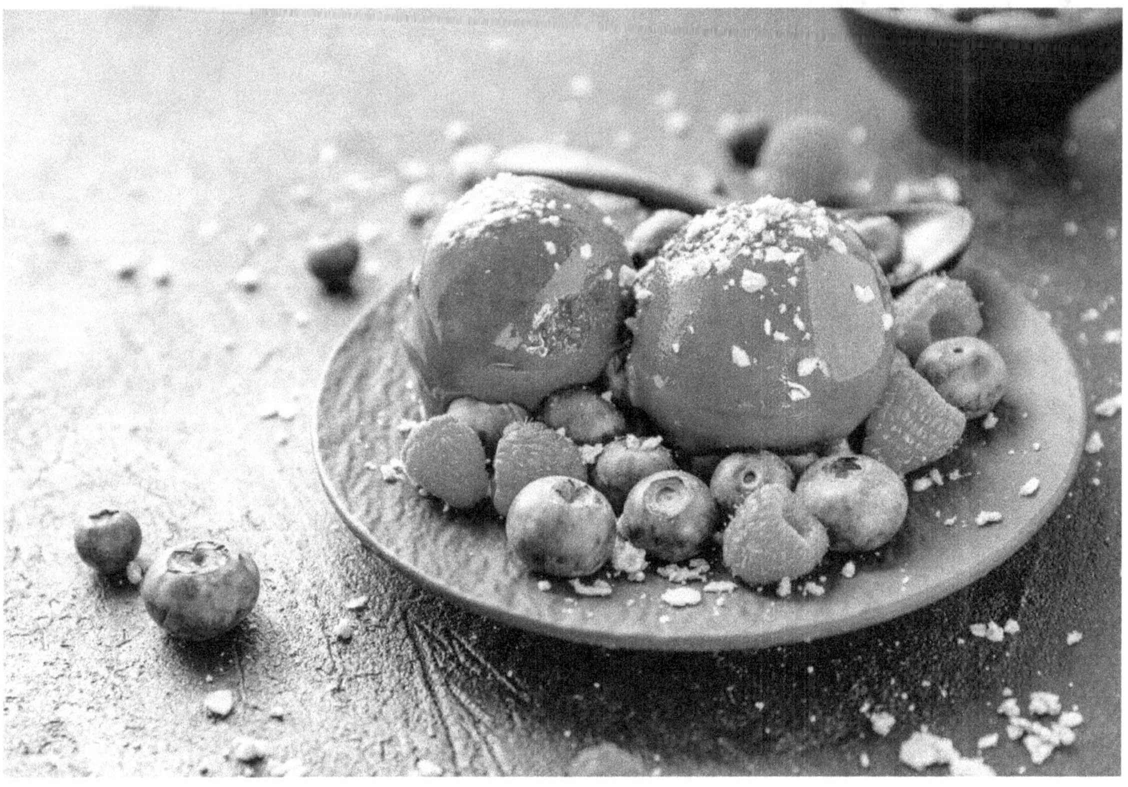

The ice cream is likely going to be your favorite. It is loaded with nutrients from just a few ingredients. Don't miss out on the strawberry and raspberry incorporated flavor.

Servings: 2

Cook time: 1 minute

Ingredients:

- 1 tbsp. chopped fresh mint
- 1 c. frozen strawberries
- 2 frozen bananas
- 1 c. frozen raspberries

Directions:

1. In a blender, blend the frozen strawberries, raspberries, and bananas on high, or on the purée setting for 30 to 60 seconds.

2. Sprinkle each serving with fresh mint.

3. Serve immediately.

Conclusion

While some memory deficits are common as you age (forgetting where you placed your keys, you won't find a word at the tip of your language), severe memory loss is not a guaranteed thing. By focusing on what you eat, you can keep your mind healthy and raise the risk of severe memory deterioration. Your diet, along with some other lifestyle factors, will influence the way your brain functions and develop your logical thinking skills such as learning something new, processing important information, addressing problems, managing complex tasks, and critically thinking.

The effect of diet on memory can be achieved surprisingly quickly. The memory will increase as quickly as 1 hour after a protein drink and go down one hour after a glucose drink. In addition, a low-glycemic breakfast (with a slight decrease in glucose after peaks) with better verbal memory in the course of the morning than a high-glycemic breakfast (with high-grade glucose peaks and rapid decreases).

Nutrition has an effect on brain function; however, well beyond the hours of consumption. Yes, for years, the food we consume may have a positive or detrimental impact on our brain health.

Early work has shown that diets in the Mediterranean and DASH have a link to better brain health, perhaps as a result of enhanced cardiovascular functioning. Researchers wondered, however, whether these results can be strengthened by mixing the most beneficial Mediterranean and DASH diets with foodstuffs known to enhance brain health and foods, which should be minimized because of their negative impact on brain health. The MIND (Mediterranean-DASH Delay Intervention) Diet was thus established. The findings of retrospective MIND Diet studies were groundbreaking.

It's not necessary — or even a good idea — to wait for signs that your memory drops until your brain health is discussed. By eating like your mind, you can maximize your brain's working and think abilities rely on this – because they do.

That said, it's always a good idea to consult with your doctor before you start a restrictive diet.

I hope you have learned something!

Author's Afterthoughts

THANK YOU

I am thankful for downloading this book and taking the time to read it. I know that you have learned a lot and you had a great time reading it. Writing books is the best way to share the skills I have with your and the best tips too.

I know that there are many books and choosing my book is amazing. I am thankful that you stopped and took time to decide. You made a great decision and I am sure that you enjoyed it.

I will be even happier if you provide honest feedback about my book. Feedbacks helped by growing and they still do. They help me to choose better content and new ideas. So, maybe your feedback can trigger an idea for my next book.

Thank you again

Sincerely

Ivy Hope